Eat to Win

The content of this book was carefully researched. However, readers should always consult a qualified medical specialist for individual advice before adopting any new nutrition plan. This book should not be used as an alternative to seeking specialist medical advice.

All information is supplied without liability. Neither the author nor the publisher will be liable for possible disadvantages, injuries, or damages.

Laura Kealy
ANutr, SENr

EAT
to
WIN

Nutrition for Peak Performance
in Female Team Sport Athletes

Fuelling • Recovery • Energy

Meyer & Meyer Sport

British Library of Cataloguing in Publication Data
A catalogue record for this book is available from the British Library

Eat to Win
Maidenhead: Meyer & Meyer Sport (UK) Ltd., 2023
ISBN: 978-1-78255-251-2

© 2023 by Meyer & Meyer Sport (UK) Ltd.
Aachen, Auckland, Beirut, Cairo, Cape Town, Dubai, Hägendorf, Hong Kong, Indianapolis, Maidenhead,
Manila, New Delhi, Singapore, Sydney, Tehran, Vienna
 Member of the World Sport Publishers' Association (WSPA), www.w-s-p-a.org
Printed by Print Consult GmbH, Munich, Germany
Printed in Slovakia

ISBN: 978-1-78255-251-2
Email: info@m-m-sports.com
www.thesportspublisher.com

Contents

Acknowledgements

This book would have remained only an idea if it were not for the encouragement, support, and guidance of many people.

To my girlfriend, Ais. Thank you for always being in my corner, for giving me the belief that I can pursue projects I deem beyond my reach, and for being my most honest recipe tester. Your endless patience, love, and support means the world to me. This book is for you.

To my parents, Brigid and Tom, and my brothers, Fergus, Niall, and Damien. You have been a constant support system for me in life. I wouldn't be where I am today without the love and unconditional encouragement you each provide. I count myself incredibly lucky to have you as family.

To Liz and Meyer & Meyer Sport, thank you for your belief in my concept and this book. For all the team's hard work, and your appreciation of the importance of the subject matter.

Thank you to Madz, Cara, and Luke for your beautiful work with my graphics and photos – you took very rough guidelines and produced work far greater than I could have imagined! A big thank you to Julie and Paul for use of their beautiful kitchen; you came to my rescue!

To all those who have helped spread the word around the world that there was finally a performance nutrition book written specifically for female team sport athletes. Thank you for the support; I hope it won't be the last book written for you.

Finally, to you, the reader. Thank you for buying this book, I hope it helps improve your sports performance, health, and happiness.

Introduction

Optimal nutrition all comes down to your daily habits. You are the sum of your repeated actions, so if you have nutritious daily eating habits, you will most likely meet all your nutrient needs. When it comes to changing and improving your diet, it is best to assess and modify how you currently eat. It can be tempting to try and completely overhaul your nutrition, but this isn't advised. Doing so will most likely make you feel restricted, and this may cause unnecessary stress for you and usually leads back to your original eating habits. My recommendation would be to try and improve your current food habits one day at a time. This way, you can make gradual changes that you are far more likely to stick to long term.

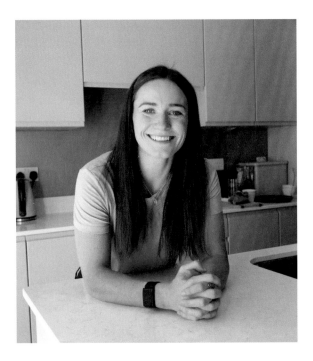

The aims of this book are simple:

- To improve your knowledge around health and performance nutrition.
- To show you that healthy cooking doesn't have to be boring or complicated.
- To teach you how to fuel adequately for training sessions and matches.
- To teach you how to refuel and recover in the time after.

Why I Wrote This Book

I've been playing team sports since I was seven. Like most girls back in the early 1990s, I played on the boys' team, and although we have now progressed to all-female teams across dozens of sports, it seems we are still treated as small men. This is due to a severe lack of research in sports nutrition and performance in girls and women. A study from 2022 concluded that only 6% of sport and exercise studies from 2014 to 2020 were conducted with only female participants (Lew, Lindsay A et al., 2022).

There is an obvious absence of female-specific nutrition recommendations in sport. This means that, just like back in the 90s, there are few resources out there for women and girls playing team sports who want to perform at their very best! I set up my business Bridge Nutrition because I have a passion for performance nutrition, and I've spent the last 8 years working with females across a range of field and court-based sports. Combining my education and experience, this book contains everything you need to know about how to eat for optimal health and to maximise your performance!

All recommendations within this book are established and evidence based. As this is a book written for individuals who may not have a background or education in nutrition, I have not included all scientific references. However, please reach out to me if you require references for any of the information provided and I will happily provide my sources.

What Is a Team Sport Athlete?

A team sport includes any sport that involves players working together towards a shared objective. It is an activity in which a group of individuals on the same team work together through athleticism and strategy to win a competitive game or match. This can be seen in sports such as soccer, hockey, rugby league, rugby union, Australian rules football, American football, Gaelic football, basketball, volleyball, cricket, camogie, lacrosse, handball and many others. Every team sport is different to some degree. However, these field and court team sports share a lot of similarities in terms of athletic requirements.

Players are required to be physically fit and strong. Games demand high-intensity repeated sprint work, with short bouts of rest in between. Players may be tackled by the opposition and, in turn, must be able to tackle; this requires a level of strength and resilience. Players have strategized playing positions and must remain mentally focused and switched on throughout matches. As decades of scientific research has proven, the nutrition choices a team sport athlete makes will have a significant impact on all the above – which is where this book comes in!

The Athlete Mindset

I work with a range of athletes at both elite and recreational levels. Players often think that just because they play at a lower division or because they don't get paid for playing, they don't have to put as much effort into their lifestyle habits, such as nutrition and sleep. Something I always make clear is that no matter what level you play at, if you are competing in a sport that requires physical strength, speed and/or endurance, you are an athlete! If you can start *considering* yourself as an athlete, you are more likely to think and *behave* like an athlete. This should help you to make food and lifestyle choices that are conducive to improving your performance.

Part I

Your Personal Nutrition and Nutrition for Performance

We need to adopt different nutritional strategies depending on our desired outcomes. Some will need to be acute (short term), and some will need to be provisional (long term). If you are looking to perform at your best for a match, then you need to fuel up appropriately via a high carbohydrate intake in the days beforehand. Conversely, if you are looking to drop body fat, then you need to adhere to a calorie deficit for a long period of time. If you are seeking optimal health, you should try to meet all your nutrient requirements via well-balanced, food-first intake. The point I'm making here, is that your food choices should be adjusted to your goals. A mistake I commonly see is athletes trying to achieve multiple goals at the same time with their nutrition (performance, body fat loss, muscle gain etc.). The usual outcome is that the player doesn't hit any of their goals and ends up fed up and frustrated at the whole process.

In this book, you will be shown how to make the right food choices for your health and athletic performance. I recommend that you focus on one goal at a time and don't try to do everything at once!

Finding the Balance Between Health and Performance

One thing to make clear from the start is that nutrition for health and nutrition for performance are not the same things. There are foods that may be recommended for performance that may not be particularly high in micronutrients. However, they may contain fast-acting carbs for energy, easily absorbed protein for recovery or may help you hit high-calorie targets.

A pitfall some athletes fall into is trying to eat only what they think are 'healthy' foods. This may lead you to avoid foods that are necessary for optimal performance and to meet specific nutrient targets. A processed, high sugar cereal bar might have little-to-no vitamins, minerals, protein or fibre, but it might be the exact thing you need to eat to help fuel a training session or match! So, throughout this book you will get the exact same advice as I give my athletes: Keep it simple, and don't overthink it!

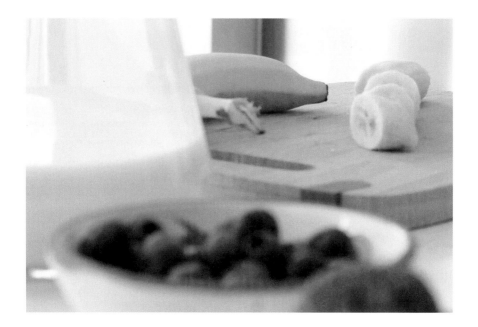

Chapter 1

Nutrition 101

Calories

Calories have often been over-complicated by mainstream media. They are demonised, feared and misunderstood. Put simply, calories are a unit of energy. The more calories a food contains, the more energy it provides.

Our bodies use the calories (energy) from our food in different ways. As you can see from the following diagram, much of our energy intake is used by our basal metabolic rate.

- *BMR*: Basal Metabolic Rate – calories burned when resting (respiration, digestion, organ function, brain function, etc.). The rate of this will depend on your body mass; this isn't something you can change.
- *TEF*: Thermic Effect of Food – the calories you burn processing the food you eat. Certain foods can increase TEF, such as a high protein diet.
- *NEAT*: Non-Exercise Activity Thermogenesis – these are the calories you burn by movement outside of exercise (walking, standing, fidgeting, cleaning, washing the car, walking up the stairs, cooking, etc.).
- *TEA*: Thermic Effect of Activity (also known as EAT: Exercise Activity Thermogenesis) – calories burned through exercise.

The following figure is a breakdown of what our body uses calories for. The biggest one (outside of BMR) is NEAT. If you move a lot outside training, you must be aware of your level of NEAT. If you do 8 km of walking or a long commute on a bike to work on top of your training session, you need to make sure you are consuming adequate calories to cover all your physical movement. To calculate your required calories, you can follow the below equation (Harris-Benedict):

$$BMR = 10 \times weight\ (kg) + 6.25 \times height\ (cm) - 5 \times age\ (years) - 161$$

CALORIES BURNED

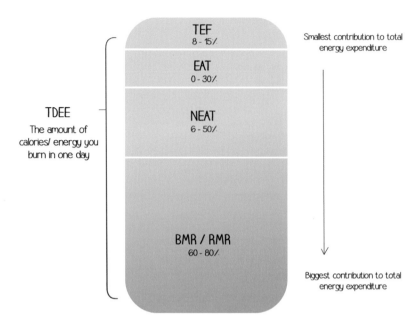

* This is a generalisation. Contributions are variable.
Individual context and situations will change contributions

To determine your total daily calorie needs, you then multiply your BMR by your physical activity level (PAL):

- Sedentary (little or no exercise): calories = BMR × 1.2
- Lightly active (light exercise/sports 1–3 days/week): calories = BMR × 1.375
- Moderately active (moderate exercise/sports 3–5 days/week): calories = BMR × 1.55
- Very active (hard exercise/sports 6–7 days a week): calories = BMR × 1.725
- If you are extra active (very hard exercise/sports and a physical job): calories = BMR × 1.9

So, let's use my friend Emma as an example. She is a 26-year-old teacher who plays football and trains four times a week. She is 168 cm and 65 kg. Her PAL is moderately active (1.55). Her calorie calculation would be as follows:

- BMR = 10 × 65 (kg) + 6.25 × 168 (cm) − 5 × 26 (years) − 161 = 1409 calories
- BMR × PAL = 1409 × 1.55 = 2183 calories

This is the minimum number of calories that Emma needs to cover her energy requirements. If her training load increases via frequency, intensity or volume, she should increase her calories accordingly.

Macronutrients

Carbohydrates, proteins and fats are called macronutrients. All food is made up of one, two or all three of these nutrients. We need these in large amounts in our diets, and the amount of each you should consume will vary depending on your desired outcomes.

We fuel our bodies with the food we eat. If we under consume one or more of these nutrients, or mainly consume lower nutrient foods, our bodies may become under-fuelled or undernourished. If this continues unaddressed, you are at risk of ill health, underperforming, injury and burnout.

Macronutrient	Calories per gram
Carbohydrates	4
Protein	4
Fat	9

Carbohydrate

Carbohydrates have had a lot of bad press over the last few years. The anti-carb movement blamed the rising rates of obesity on increased consumption of carbohydrates by the public. Low carb diets soared in popularity, and people started cutting bread, pasta and other nutritious sources of carbohydrate from their daily intake – all of which was mostly unnecessary and unsustainable.

So, let's get a couple of things straight. The macronutrient itself does not cause any negative health effects in otherwise healthy individuals. However, there are many different sources of carbohydrates, from lentils and fruit (nutrient-dense) to pizza and ice cream (nutrient sparse). Some are more nutritious and others less so.

Carbohydrates are the body's preferred primary fuel source. They provide energy to your muscles, during movement and exercise, and to the central nervous system (brain) throughout the day. If you play high-intensity repeated sprint sports (which, if you are reading this book, I presume you do!) you need to focus on carbohydrates for fuelling your training sessions and matches. Inadequate carbohydrate intake will lead to poor fuelling and refuelling and, ultimately, result in a sub-optimal performance. The following table shows the carbohydrate recommendations for athletes. You will see here that on days where you are training for about an hour you should aim for 5–7 g/kg of body weight, and on days where you are required to perform for more than an hour, you should aim for 6–10 g/kg of body weight.

Daily Carbohydrate Needs for Fuel and Recovery for Athletes

Light	Low-intensity/skills-based activities	3–5 g/kg of body weight/day
Moderate	Moderate exercise programme (e.g., 1 h per day)	5–7 g/kg of body weight/day
High	Endurance programme (e.g., 1–3 h per day, moderate-high intensity)	6–10 g/kg of body weight/day
Very High	Extreme Commitment (e.g., 4–5 h per day, moderate-high intensity)	8–12 g/kg of body weight/day

That means on training days, depending on your weight, you should be aiming for a minimum of the below carbohydrate intake:

- 55 kg: 5 × 55 = 275 g
- 60 kg: 5 × 60 = 300 g
- 65 kg: 5 × 65 = 325 g
- 70 kg: 5 × 70 = 350 g
- 75 kg: 5 × 75 = 375 g

You can use the recipes in this book to help you reach these high carbohydrate targets. If you focus on high carb meals and snacks throughout the day, you will find it easier to follow this well-proven advice.

Snacks	Carbohydrates (g)
30 g bag of popcorn	25 g
Cereal bar	30 g
50 g of granola	30 g
Large bowl of cereal and milk	80 g
3 rice cakes	20 g
20 g dried fruit	20 g
3 Jaffa cakes	24 g
4 cream crackers	18 g
500 mL isotonic sports drink	30 g
2 slices of white toast and jam	40 g
20 g of jellies	15 g

There are two main types of carbs:

1. Slow-releasing (starchy/complex) carbohydrates

We want to focus on slow-releasing carbs for most of our intake to ensure we keep our blood sugars stable and have a constant release of energy throughout the day. They take longer to digest and therefore result in a steady release of energy throughout the hours after. These complex carbohydrates are often a good source of fibre as well (more to come on that in the next section). Once consumed, carbs are broken down to glucose, which is their simplest form, and then stored as glycogen in our muscles and liver. This stored glycogen is used during periods where there is an energy demand from your body, i.e. movement or exercise. It is this stored glycogen that will be used during your training sessions or games. The longer the duration or the higher the intensity of the exercise, the more glycogen required to fuel the session. Therefore, optimal carbohydrate intake is key to performing at your best. Optimal carb consumption means optimal performance.

2. Fast-releasing (sugary/simple) carbohydrates

These types of carbohydrates are quickly broken down and absorbed by the body. They usually result in a quick spike in blood sugars and subsequent increase in energy levels. Unfortunately, this increase in energy is short-lived; and if more energy isn't consumed, it is usually followed by a drop in blood sugar levels, which leads to low energy levels. If you predominately consume simple, sugary carbohydrates throughout the day, you may experience periods of short bursts of high energy followed by spells of low energy and fatigue. For this reason, we want to avoid relying on sugary carbs for our energy intake. However, at certain times, when we are aiming to perform at our best, consuming fast-acting sugary carbs will be to our advantage (this is covered in chapter 3).

Fibre

Fibre is so important that it gets its own section! It is vital to numerous aspects of health, including heart and gastrointestinal health. Fibre is made up of the parts of plants that we cannot digest, which pass, mostly unchanged, through our digestive system.

Types of Fibre

There are two types of fibre: soluble and insoluble. Soluble fibre dissolves in water and helps control blood sugar levels and reduce cholesterol. Good sources include beans, oats, oat bran, rice bran, citrus fruits, apples, strawberries, peas, barley and potatoes. Insoluble fibre does not dissolve in water. It is bulky and helps to prevent constipation. This kind of fibre is found in whole grains (which is why we choose whole grain bread, pasta, rice, noodles, etc. over the white variety), wheat cereals, nuts and seeds, fruit and vegetable skins, and vegetables such as corn, aubergine (eggplant), green beans, broccoli, spinach and kale.

How Much Do We Need?

The recommended adult daily intake for health benefits is approximately 30 g. However, with the world going crazy for gluten free and low carb diets, we simply don't get enough daily fibre (on average about 15–17 g).

How Do You Know If You're Getting Enough?

A good sign that you don't have enough fibre in your diet is constipation and bloating. Now there are other things that may cause constipation, but your fibre intake is a good place to start. Conversely, going from eating little fibre to overloading on high fibre food isn't recommended either, as too much fibre can cause bloating, gas and pain. So up your intake gradually to the recommended 30 g.

Benefits

A high fibre diet has a host of health benefits, including lower risk of heart disease, lower risk of diabetes, lower risk of certain cancers, improved skin health, improved digestive health and can also help with weight loss. Ultimately, if you want to perform at your best on the pitch or court and keep energised throughout the day, you need to see carbohydrates as an important weapon in your health and performance nutrition arsenal.

Protein

The importance of protein seems to be well accepted among team sport athletes, with the use of protein supplements and foods skyrocketing in recent years. Protein is an essential nutrient, and although it may be only thought of in relation to muscle building, it is responsible for multiple physiological functions. Protein is the foundation for tissues, organs, cells, skin and muscles. This macronutrient also makes up enzymes, hormones and antibodies. At least 10,000 different proteins make you what you are and keep you that way. When protein is consumed, it is broken down in the stomach into amino acids. These amino acids are then absorbed into the bloodstream by the small intestine. There are 20 amino acids, and our bodies make them in two different ways: either from scratch or by manipulating other amino acids. Nine of the 20 amino acids are known as *essential amino acids* (EAA). We cannot

Essential Amino Acid	Nonessential Amino Acid
Isoleucine	Alanine
Leucine	Arginine
Lysine	Asparagine
Methionine	Aspartic acid
Phenylalanine	Cysteine
Threonine	Glutamic acid
Tryptophan	Glutamine
Valine	Glycine
	Proline
	Serine
	Tyrosine

make these EAAs and so we must obtain them from food. When absorbed, these amino acids will form polymers (a chain-like structure), which will, in turn, form proteins. The newly formed proteins will then go on to serve a particular function within the body. These functions range from the formation of muscle cells, muscle fibres, energy production, enzymes and cell structure.

When it comes to muscle growth, there is one EAA that is particularly important: leucine. Research has shown that there is likely a leucine threshold that must be passed to stimulate muscle protein synthesis (MPS); this is thought to be 2–3 g of leucine per meal. Consuming protein-based foods high in leucine means you will have greater muscle repair and growth. Food high in leucine include dairy, chicken breast, lean beef, tinned tuna, salmon, turkey breast, eggs, corn, wheat and soy. Everyone needs protein in their diet, but as an athlete, you will require a higher protein intake to repair and rebuild skeletal muscle and connective tissues following intense training sessions and games. For the general population, the recommendation is about 0.8–1 g/kg body weight (BW). For team sport players, the recommendation is 1.6–2 g/kg BW.

Body Weight (kg)	Protein Target (g) (1.6–2 g/kg BW)
55	88–110
65	104–130
75	120–150
85	136–170

Your protein intake should be spread across your day for a more sustained delivery of amino acids to the body. This is due to the dose-dependent relationship between protein intake and MPS. Ideally, your daily protein would look something like this:

Meal/Snack	Protein (g) 110–170 g
Breakfast	20–30
Mid-Morning Snack	10–20
Lunch	30–40
Mid-Afternoon Snack	10–20
Dinner	30–40
Evening Snack	10–20

Animal-Based Foods	30 g of Protein	Plant-Based Foods	30 g of Protein
Eggs	4	Chickpeas (tinned)	400 g
Salmon (uncooked)	150 g	Kidney beans (tinned)	340 g
Chicken breast (uncooked)	120 g	Baked beans (tinned)	600 g
Turkey breast (uncooked)	120 g	Mixed nuts	500 g
Cottage cheese	250 g	Peanut butter	110 g
Greek yogurt	300 g	Edamame beans (tinned)	280 g
Minced beef (uncooked)	150 g	Tofu	360 g
Cod (uncooked)	170 g	Quorn	240 g
Skimmed milk	900 mL	Soy milk	1.1 L
Cheddar cheese	120 g	Quinoa (uncooked)	220 g

Fat

When it comes to fat in our diet, we must appreciate that not all fats are created equal. Some are incredibly nutritious and vital for our health. Others should be consumed minimally as they can cause adverse effects if over consumed for a prolonged period. Fat, much like carbohydrates and protein, is an essential nutrient. Your body needs fat for energy, to absorb vitamins, for insulation and to protect your heart, brain and other vital organs. They also act as messengers, helping proteins carry out their role around the body, and are responsible for chemical reactions that control immune function, reproduction, growth, and other areas of metabolism. There are two main types of fat: saturated and unsaturated. Most fat sources contain both types in different amounts.

Saturated fats, in comparison with unsaturated fats, impact health negatively by raising low-density lipoprotein (LDL) (bad) cholesterol levels. High LDL levels put you at risk of heart attack, stroke and other major health problems. Saturated fats are best consumed in moderation. Foods containing large amounts of saturated fat include red meat, butter, cheese, cakes, biscuits, processed meats (sausages, bacon), pastries, chocolate and ice cream. Some plant-based fats, such as coconut oil and palm oil, are also rich in saturated fat.

Unsaturated fats (known as healthy, or essential fats) are subdivided into monounsaturated and polyunsaturated fats. They help lower risk of cardiovascular disease and overall mortality. Foods high in unsaturated fats include vegetable oils (such as olive, canola, sunflower, soy and corn), avocado, most nuts, most seeds and oily fish. You should try to include sources of these healthy fats in your daily diet. See images in chapter 2 for sample portion sizes.

Micronutrients

Vitamins and minerals are essential nutrients that your body needs in small amounts to function optimally. A balanced diet usually provides all the essential vitamins and minerals you need. There are a couple of exceptions, and I will talk about those more in the supplements section in chapter 3.

Minerals

Minerals are vital for your body to stay healthy. Your body uses minerals for many different jobs, including keeping your bones, muscles, heart and brain healthy. Minerals are also important for making enzymes and hormones. The following table shows the most important ones to know and where to find them in the diet.

Mineral	Function	Found in
Iron	Part of a molecule (haemoglobin) found in red blood cells that carries oxygen in the body, needed for energy metabolism.	Organ meats, red meats, fish, poultry, shellfish, egg yolks, legumes, dried fruit, dark, leafy greens, iron-fortified breads and breakfast cereals.
Zinc	Cell growth, creation of DNA, building proteins, damaged tissue, repair and supporting a healthy immune system.	Meat, fish, poultry, whole grains and vegetables.

Mineral	Function	Found in
Iodine	Needed to make thyroid hormones. These hormones control the body's metabolism and many other important functions.	Cod, tuna, dairy products and shellfish
Potassium	Needed for proper fluid balance, nerve transmission and muscle contraction.	Meat, milk, fresh fruit and vegetables, whole grains and legumes.
Calcium	Important for healthy bones and teeth, muscle contraction, nerve function, blood clotting, blood pressure regulation and immune system health.	Milk and milk products, canned fish with bones (salmon, sardines), fortified tofu and fortified soymilk, greens (broccoli, mustard greens), legumes.
Magnesium	Needed for making protein, muscle contraction, nerve transmission, immune system health.	Nuts and seeds, legumes, leafy green vegetables, seafood, chocolate, and artichokes.

Vitamins

Vitamins are organic substances required by your body to maintain optimal health. Vitamins can be water-soluble or fat-soluble. Water-soluble vitamins are packed into the watery portion of the foods you eat. They are absorbed directly into the bloodstream as food is broken down during digestion or as a supplement. Fat-soluble vitamins are present in foods containing fats, and your body absorbs these vitamins as it does dietary fats.

Vitamin	Function	Found in
Water-Soluble		
C	Plays important roles in immune system function. It is also an antioxidant, which helps counteract oxidative stress caused by exercise.	Orange juice, cherries, red peppers, kale, grapefruit and green leafy veg.
B complex	B vitamins help release energy from food. Thiamine, riboflavin, niacin, pantothenic acid and biotin engage in energy production. Vitamins B6, B12 and folic acid metabolise amino acids and help cells multiply.	Whole grains, meat, eggs, dairy products, legumes, seeds, nuts, leafy green veg and fruit.

(continued)

(continued)

Vitamin	Function	Found in
Fat-Soluble		
A	Healthy eyes and general growth and development, including healthy teeth and skin.	Carrots and other orange foods, including sweet potato and cantaloupe melons, liver and spinach.
D	Assists with absorption of calcium, immune function and wound healing.	Eggs, fish and mushrooms.
E	Blood circulation and protection from free radicals.	Nuts (especially almonds), sunflower seeds and tomatoes.
K	Helps to make proteins needed for blood clotting and the building of bones.	Leafy greens, such as kale, spinach, Brussels sprouts and broccoli.

Hydration

Adequate fluid intake is essential for both health and performance. Even slight dehydration can slow us both physically and mentally. Aim to drink at least 35 mL per kg of body weight. Your urine is a very good indicator of your hydration status. Aim for a pale-yellow colour, and check every time you go to the toilet. The figure on the next page shows examples of your level of hydration based on your urine colour. Begin hydrating as soon as you wake up in the morning; many of us will skip fluids in the earlier part of the day and spend the rest of it in a dehydrated state! Keep a bottle of water by your bed and take a few sips when your alarm goes off in the morning and keep drinking it as you are getting ready.

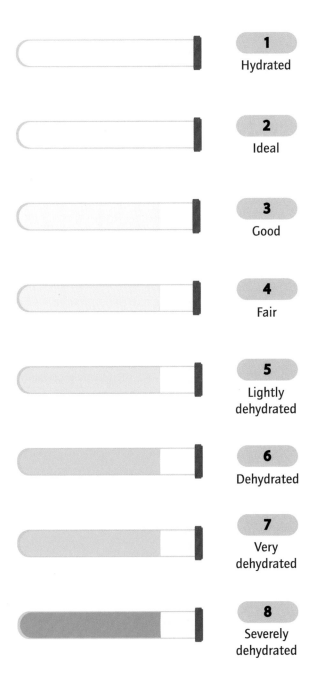

Chapter 2

Nutrition for Health

How to Build a Balanced Meal

Our main meals throughout the day – breakfast, lunch and dinner – are great opportunities to meet our nutrient requirements. When putting a meal together, the aim is to include foods that cover your main nutritional needs, such as our macro- and micronutrients (covered in chapter 1). If you can build balanced, nutrient-dense meals, you will give yourself the best chance of ensuring you have a healthy diet.

While it is not compulsory to eat breakfast to be healthy, most find that starting the day with a healthy, balanced meal can set them up for better food choices for the rest of the day. If you have a high training load, then I would certainly recommend breakfast. If you struggle to eat early in the day, then try to have a smoothie (chapter 11), which should be easier to consume than a full meal. Aim to hit all four of the following groups and you will start your day the right way.

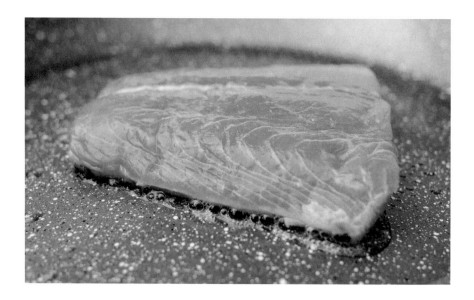

Here is an easy blueprint to help you create balanced meals. Pick something from each of the four nutrient pillars:

1. **Complex carbs:** These are slow-releasing carbs and will keep you feeling fuller for longer, keep energy levels high throughout the day and add some fibre to each of your meals.
2. **Protein:** We now know how important protein is and if you are aiming for a high intake, ensure you have a decent amount of protein with each meal (20–40 g).
3. **Healthy fats:** Add some fat to each meal to meet your requirements. Remember, our bodies need some fat for energy, to absorb vitamins and to protect your heart and brain health.
4. **Fruit/Veg:** I recommend 3+ portions of fruit per day and 4+ portions of veg for active players training several times a week and competing. While it's easy to snack on fruit, vegetables can be a bit trickier. Include a minimum of two fistfuls of a variety of veg with lunch and dinner to help meet these targets.

The table on the next page shows how, with the right food choices, you can meet these four nutrient pillars with main meals.

Portion Sizes

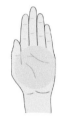

A serving of protein = 1 palm

A serving of vegetables = 1 fist

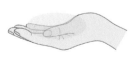

A serving of carbs = 1 cupped hand

A serving of fats = 1 thumb

To avoid going down the path of weighing your food, you can use your hand to measure out portion sizes of different types of food. This is a rough system of measurement but will ensure you are getting an adequate amount of each food type (and their required nutrients!) It may also help if you are concerned about over- or under-eating certain foods. Please note, this form of measurement is a rough guide, and although it won't be accurate to the gram, it will give you a good shot at hitting your macro- and micronutrient needs.

	Complex Carbs	Protein	Fat	Fruit/ Veg
Breakfast – Egg and Avo Toast				
Wholegrain toast	✓			
Two Eggs		✓		
Avocado			✓	✓
Tomato				✓
Spinach				✓
Lunch – Pesto Chicken Pasta				
Whole wheat pasta	✓			
Chicken		✓		
Pesto			✓	
Pine nuts			✓	
Peppers				✓
Mushrooms				✓
Onion				✓
Dinner – All the Spuds Fish Pie				
Sweet Potato	✓			
Potato	✓			
Mixed Seafood		✓	✓	
Broccoli				✓
Carrots				✓
Peas				✓

The Non-Negotiables

At the start of every week, you should take a few minutes to consider what you want to achieve in the days ahead. Non-negotiables refer to the small habits that we do each day, no matter what. Examples of these could be your morning coffee, brushing your teeth, checking your Instagram, walking the dog, checking the news headlines, having a couple of biscuits with your 11 a.m. tea, etc. Non-negotiable habits can be considered healthy, less healthy or unhealthy. They make up our daily routine and, if we can improve them a little at a time, the accumulative effect of doing so can have major impacts on our overall health and wellbeing.

Questions to help you build your non-negotiables:

* What areas of your health do you think you need to work on?
* What are the habits you want to improve?
* What is your training schedule for the week?
* What do you need to have organised to ensure you are prepped for training so you can fuel and recover optimally?
* Do you have a game?

Examples of non-negotiables to try and build:

* Drinking at least 2 L of water a day.
* Planning training day meals and snacks in advance.
* Getting to bed at 10 p.m. every night.
* Reading 10 pages of a book each day.
* Eating four portions of vegetables every day.
* Trying to cook a new recipe once a week.

Chapter 3

Nutrition for Performance

Preseason

Most preseason training will be focused on improving strength, conditioning and fitness before the competitive season begins. You will be moving from a period of rest and reduced physical activity (off season) to a more active one. This places stress on your body, and if you don't focus on your nutrition, you will not only see slow progress but may also increase your risk of injury and illness.

If your preseason goal is an increase of strength and muscle gain, you must incorporate several daily habits to stimulate MPS successfully. A calorie surplus, adequate protein, optimal sleep, adequate nutrient intake, resistance training, progressive overload, hydration and optimal protein distribution are daily habits that need to be built over a long period of time to gain significant mass. When you have built these habits and are confident you are going in the right direction, you can introduce other strategies, such as creatine, to help with progression (discussed later in the chapter).

For low-intensity strength training and conditioning, I would recommend following the 'Recovery Day' recipes (chapter 9). These recipes are nutrient-dense, contain high amounts of protein, healthy fats, fibre and lots of veggies for additional micronutrients. For high-intensity days or days with double training sessions, you must fuel and recover accordingly, this is covered in the next section.

In Season

Nutrition throughout your competitive season should focus around fuelling and recovering optimally for your training sessions and competitive games. In team sports, a player is required to have repeated sprint ability, strength to tackle and retain possession, and to recover efficiently in between plays. The food and drink you consume on a training or game day will have a direct impact on how well you train or play, and if the right pre-exercise nutrition can give you the edge, then why would you overlook it?

A practical way to remember how to fuel correctly is to follow the five Fs of fuelling:

1. Food

Carbs are essential and are our body's main source of fuel for high-intensity exercise. Fuelling correctly before exercise can help sustain energy, boost performance, preserve muscle mass and speed up recovery. A total of 1–1.5 g/kg BW of carbohydrates about 1.5–3 hours before the workout should be adequate, e.g. a 65 kg athlete would aim for 65–98 g of carbohydrates. On high-intensity training days, you require a large amount of complex (starchy) carbohydrates. These include pasta, rice, noodles, oats, lentils, quinoa, bread, pitta breads, bagels, wraps, potatoes and sweet potatoes.

2. Fruit

Fruit is a fantastic source of carbohydrates, so mix it up!

- 1 cup pineapple = 22 g
- 1 medium pear = 27 g
- 1 medium banana = 27 g
- 1 medium apple = 25 g
- 1 cup grapes = 27 g

3. Frequency

Four to six hours before exercising, your main meal should be made up of a large amount of complex carbohydrates (slow-release energy). Then a large snack/small meal 2–3 hours before, made up of easily absorbed carbohydrates (quick-releasing energy). Then 30–60 mins before exercising, you should top up with a liquid or very easily absorbed carb-based snack (sports drink, jellies, fruit, cereal bar, Jaffa cakes, rice cakes, dried fruit or carb gels).

4. Fluid

Dehydration of only 2% can decrease brain, muscle and organ function, while also reducing sports and exercise performance. Aim for 35 mL/kg BW per day (a 65 kg athlete would aim for about 2.275 L). Consume 500 mL of fluid in the 2 hours before training. Milk, tea, coffee, fruit juices, soups and smoothies all contribute to your fluid intake. Aim for a pale-yellow colour for your urine – this is a good indicator of hydration.

5. Forbidden – Fiery, Fried, Fat, Fibre

Certain food types can slow down the absorption of carbs and can cause gastrointestinal discomfort. These include high fibre foods, foods with high fat content, spicy foods and deep-fried food. Try to avoid these foods within 3–4 hours before exercise.

Your training type, duration and intensity should dictate how many carbs you should aim for. Fuelling for the work required is a strategy that involves adapting your carbohydrate intake to match your training load. In the diagram, you can see I've used the simple example of a dinner plate and advised different amounts of carbs depending on the type of day it is.

On high training or match days, you should aim to fill half of a large plate with complex (starchy) carbohydrates. These include pasta, rice, couscous, noodles, oats, lentils, quinoa, bread, pitta breads, bagels, wraps, potatoes, sweet potatoes, beans, chickpeas, etc. These types of food are high in carbohydrates, which, when eaten, are stored as glycogen in your muscles and liver. It is then used to fuel your body during moderate-to-high intensity exercise.

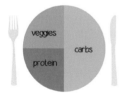 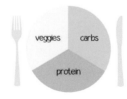 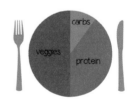

The rest of the plate should be vegetables/fruit and protein sources. Opt for lean sources of protein, such as chicken, turkey or fish. Lean red meat is a good option once a week to increase haem iron. Try and get as many different varieties of fruit and vegetables in as you can. Remember, there's nothing wrong with frozen veg or tinned options if fresh veg isn't available. On higher training or match days, we can reduce our vegetable and protein portions with our main meals to allow for an increased complex carbohydrates intake.

On moderate training days, where we don't need as much fuel, we can do a three-way split between carbs, protein and fruit/veg. I would recommend this type of day for low-intensity exercise and gym sessions.

On rest and recovery days, we can reduce those complex carbs down again and really focus on our protein and fruit/veg intake. Please be aware that if your rest day is sandwiched between two training days, you should opt for the moderate training day advice to ensure you are fully refuelled for the following day.

Nutrient Timing – Fuelling

Timing your meals and snacks appropriately on practice and game days can ensure you are fully fuelled and prepared. It can also help avoid food-related stitches or cramps. I like to get my athletes to follow the 6-3-1 rule. This is a handy way to remember what times you should try to eat at in the lead-up to the training or match:

* Six hours out – last large carbohydrate-based meal
* Three hours out – last large carbohydrate-based snack
* One hour out – last small carbohydrate-based snack

Aim to have a larger amount of complex carbohydrates 4–6 hours before the session and a large, simple carb-based snack about 3 hours out from the session. If you are aiming for your best possible performance or know that you are in for a tough session, aim for about 1.5 g/kg of carbs about 3 hours before your workout/training/match. For a 70 kg player, this would be about 70–105 g of carbs. This can be broken down into a couple of snacks, a light meal or a combination of both.

You need to figure out how much you can tolerate in the 1–3 hours before your workout. Some people can eat right before they train, and others need to avoid it. Never try anything new before a competition or match. Your nutrition strategy should be perfected on training days; work out what food works for you and what time suits you best.

Pre-exercise meals should be high in complex carbohydrates, such as porridge (oatmeal), potatoes, pasta, rice, quinoa, couscous, etc. As you get closer to the training session start time, focus on easily absorbed, simple carbohydrates, such as fruit, low-fat yogurt, granola, fruit juices, dried fruit, cereal, biscuit bars, etc. You must also ensure you are hydrated. Check your urine colour throughout the day as a good indicator (aim for a pale-yellow colour).

Nutrient Timing – Recovery

With hard training sessions exhausting fuel stores and breaking down muscle tissue, it is also vital that you have adequate carbohydrates and protein after training. Focus on the five Rs of recovery:

1. Rehydrate

Replacement of 150% of fluid losses incurred during exercise is recommended (1.5 L for every 1 kg lost during training) within the first 1–3 hours after your finish. Opt for a fluid with carbs and electrolytes for enhanced rehydration. Options: water, low-fat milk, sports drink, fruit juice.

2. Refuel

Refuel with carbohydrates to give your body the energy it needs to recover and adapt to the training session. Total carb requirement post-exercise is determined by the intensity and the duration of your session. Options: sports drink, low-fat milk, fruit juice, fruit, cereal bars, cereal and milk, low-fat yogurt, quark, bread, pasta, rice, beans, popcorn, rice cakes, potatoes, lentils, quinoa, porridge.

3. Repair

Exercise causes damage to tissue. To help tissues repair and stimulate MPS, post-workout nutrition should also include a good quality source of protein. Options: low-fat milk, yogurt, tuna, chicken, protein shake, beans, eggs, fish, turkey, lean steak, Quorn, tofu.

4. Replenish

Replenish with nutrient-rich foods loaded with vitamins and minerals to help reinforce your immune system. Plant-based foods are rich in micronutrients, antioxidants and other important compounds for health and performance. Options: berries, green leafy veg, apples, pears, banana, beans, grapes, oranges, kiwis, peas, lentils, carrots, beetroot, broccoli, nuts, seeds, tomatoes, pepper (or any fruit and veg really – the more variety, the better!)

5. Rest

Aim for a decent night's sleep, avoid alcohol. Rest is not only important for recovery but also for growth and keeping your immune system strong. Get to bed as early as you can.

You should then have a carb- and protein-based meal shortly after that to ensure you give your body the food it needs to repair and refuel itself. Don't stress too much if you can't get something to eat immediately after you finish – you won't undo your training or anything like that, but if you can start recovering right away, why wait?!

I have devised a sample training day meal plan for a 65 kg player (please note that this is not a standard weight, it's just for sample purposes). These meal plans are created using the recipes from this book and you can swap in recipes as you please as they all have full nutrient information.

- Carb recommendations are based on a 65 kg player aiming to hit a minimum of 5 g of carbohydrate per kg/BW = 325 g
- Protein recommendations are based on a 65 kg player aiming to hit approximately 2 g of protein per kg/BW = 130 g

Implementing eating strategies like these around your training session will give you the best chance of improving your performance, avoiding injury and keeping your immune system in optimal working order!

Sample Day 1 – Training at 7 p.m.

	8 a.m.	Breakfast: Loaded Porridge
	11 a.m.	Snack: Four rice cakes topped with peanut butter and banana
	2 p.m.	Lunch: Sun-dried Tomato Pesto Pasta
	4 p.m.	Fuelling snack: Low-fat yogurt with granola and an apple
	6 p.m.	Fuelling snack: Granola bar
	7–8.30 p.m.	Training
	8.30 p.m.	Post-training snack: 500 mL of chocolate milk and a banana
	9.00 p.m.	Post-training dinner: Ham and Pea Risotto

Sample Day 2 – Training 5 p.m.

	8 a.m.	Breakfast: Giddy Up Granola and Yogurt
	10 a.m.	Snack: Four oatcakes with sliced apple and almond butter
	12 p.m.	Lunch: Mexican Chicken and Quinoa
	3 p.m.	Pre-exercise snack: Berry Fuel Smoothie
	4 p.m.	Fuelling snack: Handful of dried apricots
	5–6.30 p.m.	Training
	6.30 p.m.	Post-training snack: 300 g low-fat yogurt with granola and a handful of raisins
	8.30 p.m.	Post-training dinner: Prawn Massaman Curry

Game Day Nutrition

Whatever sport you play, competitive games require you to perform at your absolute best, and your nutrition in the days leading up to the match can have a significant impact on how well you play.

Game day prep starts in the days beforehand. During this period, we should aim to consume high amounts of carbohydrates, fluids and get adequate rest. In the 36–48 hours pre-match, you should aim for 6–8 high carb meals. A nice way to remember this is *6–8 in 36–48*. This would mean that if your game is 1 p.m. on a Saturday your fuelling for it really starts on Thursday at lunch time. Thursday's lunch, and every meal, thereafter, should be a high carb meal. On top of that then you should focus on high carb snacks in between.

On match day itself, you can follow the training day examples for meal and snack types and timings. If your match is very early in the morning, then you will have a very small fuelling window. I recommend that you have an additional high carb meal the night before, as late as you comfortably can. This will help your pre-match fuelling for the next morning.

Sample Day 1 – Match at 12 p.m.

	8 a.m.	Fuelling breakfast: Wheety Banana Breakfast
	10 a.m.	Fuelling snack: Berry Fuel Smoothie
	11 a.m.	Fuelling snack: Cereal bar and handful of jelly sweets
	12–2 p.m.	Game
	2.30 p.m.	Recovery snack: 300 g low-fat yogurt with granola and handful of raisins
	3.30 p.m.	Recovery meal: Prawn Massaman Curry

Sample Day 2 – Match at 7 p.m.

	8 a.m.	Fuelling breakfast: Loaded Porridge and Mango Fuel Smoothie
	11 a.m.	Fuelling snack: 4 rice cakes topped with peanut butter and banana
	2 p.m.	Fuelling meal: Sun-dried Tomato Pesto Pasta
	4 p.m.	Fuelling snack: Low-fat yogurt with granola and an apple
	6 p.m.	Fuelling snack: Granola bar and 4 Jaffa cakes
	7–9 p.m.	Game
	9.30 p.m.	Recovery snack: 500 mL of chocolate milk and a banana
	10.00 p.m.	Recovery meal: Ham and Pea Risotto

Nutrition Strategies for Injury Rehabilitation

Players want to actively avoid injury during the playing season, however, regrettably, injury is regularly part of playing the game! While injuries are often random, unfortunate, and can vary by sport, age, level of competition, fitness and support structure, research shows that females tend to injure their pelvic/hip and/or knee joints more so than males. The most common injuries in female athletes include knee injuries and stress fractures – it is reported that women and girls are at particularly high risk for anterior cruciate ligament injuries with rates three to six times than in men (Zumwalt, 2018). There is some emerging research that links an increased risk of injury with specific phases of the menstrual cycle, however, these studies are in their infancy and, currently, we cannot conclude whether specific training should be tailored around the menstrual cycle (Herzberg et al., 2017).

There are several concerns when dealing with injury, the key ones include muscle atrophy (loss), reduced MPS, loss of strength and speed and the potential development of anabolic resistance. As well as physical rehabilitation, the athlete should focus on nutrition strategies to ensure they recover optimally. Adequate nutrition protocols are crucial for optimal recovery from injury. The following points cover the main areas that you should focus on.

* Energy Intake – Calorie balance is key. Eat as you would normally on a rest day. Avoid going into calorie deficits as this will place more stress on the injured body.
* Protein Intake – Aim for a minimum of 2 g/kg/BW daily, focusing on animal protein sources with a high leucine content.
* Nutrient-Dense Foods – Focus on adequate carbs (wholegrains, potatoes, fruit, veg, legumes), omega 3 (oily fish), iron (red meat, lentils, nuts), antioxidants (whole fruits, berries and veg).
* Sleep – Prioritise sleep (8+ hours a night). Repair hormones (HGH) are released at night, which are vital for muscle, ligament, and tendon repair. Inadequate sleep = longer recovery time.
* Hydration – Water is an essential nutrient and muscle tissue is 70%–75% water; dehydration can lead to fatigue, false hunger, and disrupted sleep.
* Supplements – When the above is prioritised you can then include some supplements to help aid recovery further: vitamin D, omega 3s, creatine, collagen and vitamin C, tart cherry juice.

- Alcohol – Alcohol negatively affects sleep and MPS. It can increase the severity of an injury and can negatively impact the rate and outcome of recovery.
- Adherence and Consistency – Recovery from an injury takes time, and to see the beneficial impact from the above strategies, you must be patient and consistent.

Some supplements may help, but you need to focus on a food-first approach before you consider them. First and foremost, you need to ensure you are consuming a nutrient-dense diet, meeting your maintenance calories, meeting protein targets, and hydrating adequately.

Chapter 4 covers the importance of sleep for athletes, but I will highlight now that sleep is imperative to your recovery if you are injured. This may mean that you need to spend 9 or 10 hours in bed. Our bodies recover and repair while we are asleep. The less sleep you get, the longer your return to play will be. Alcohol will only delay your recovery; injured players may use an injury as an excuse to cut loose and drink more than they usually would. Alcohol is a toxin and causes stress and inflammation when our bodies break it down. It disrupts sleep quality and quantity, causes dehydration, reduces MPS, and compromises your immune system. If you want your body to focus on repairing your injury, don't give it an extra job by having to deal with nights out on the town as well! Recovery time will depend on the extent of your injury but adhering to an adequate nutrition strategy consistently throughout your recovery, in tandem with your physical rehabilitation, will ensure you are doing so from both the inside and out.

Supplements

With a well-balanced diet, there is no need to take supplements for your health. Focus on a food-first approach to hit your vitamin and mineral needs. Health supplements can be expensive and, in most times, unnecessary and virtually useless. However, there are two supplements that I will recommend, the first being vitamin D. If you live in a country that doesn't get a lot of sunshine during the winter months you may be a risk of low levels of vitamin D. Low intake of oily fish is common in western society and an omega-3 supplement is also recommended. However, if you are confident that you get 1–2 portions of oily fish a week then it may not be necessary.

Supplements for Athletic Performance

The supplement industry is worth billions of euros, and the reason why is simple – it makes you think whatever they're selling will improve you to some degree. However, the fact of the matter is that most supplements out there either completely exaggerate their claims or simply don't work at all. We should always aim for a food-first approach when meeting our nutrient needs. This is not only a more balanced way to approach your nutrition, but it will also be a lot healthier for your bank account! In saying that, when you are confident you are meeting the nutrient recommendations outlined so far in this book, then you can look to certain safe, effective supplements to potentially improve your performance further. If you are an athlete subjected to drug testing, you must ensure you are only buying batch-tested or Informed Sport certified products. This means that products are subject to batch testing and can be traced if needed. A list of supplements follows with proven, safe, ergogenic effects recommended for team sport athletes:

Creatine

Creatine is one of the most well researched supplements proven to improve performance.

- What is it?
  - » Creatine is found in meat and fish, but you would need to eat huge amounts for the performance-enhancing effect, which is why we supplement with it.

- What does it do?
  - » Supplementation boosts the amount of creatine in our cells, which helps the production of adenosine triphosphate (ATP, energy). This results in the body being able for more instant bursts of power, thus enhancing your short-burst sprint, jump, kick, tackle, etc.
  - » It also has several other proven benefits, including muscle growth, improvement in cognitive function, reduction of fatigue, recovery enhancement, reduction of cramp when exercising, improvement in repeated sprint ability.

- Dose:
  - » Take 20 g (4 × 5 g) a day for 7 days (this is called the loading phase) to increase the amount of creatine in your cells, and take 5 g a day thereafter for as long as you want the effects to last. The loading phase

isn't compulsory, but it will take longer to see the performance-enhancing effects if you skip it. During the loading phase, spread the four doses of creatine throughout the day.

- What type?
  - » There are many types on the market but stick to creatine monohydrate, no others have proven to be more effective, and this is the cheapest.

Caffeine

Commonly found in our beloved coffee, caffeine can be an incredibly effective performance enhancer.

- What is it?
  - » Caffeine is both a nutrient and a drug. It is naturally occurring and found in several plants. It is found in coffee, tea, cola, cocoa, guarana, yerba mate tea and many other products.

- What does it do?
  - » Supplementation with caffeine stimulates the central nervous system (CNS), and this is the main mechanism for its ergogenic effect. Caffeine does this by binding to adenosine receptors. Adenosine usually works to depress CNS function. However, when you consume caffeine, it blocks adenosine receptors, which consequently stimulates CNS function as opposed to depressing it.

- Dose:
  - » The dose recommended for athletes is 3–6 mg/kg/BW. For a 70 kg athlete, this would be a 210–420 mg dose.

- What type?
  - » There are several different forms by which you can ingest caffeine, including coffee, tablets, gum, powder, bars and energy drinks. While all these forms have performance-enhancing effects, there is a delay of at least 20–30 minutes until they are noticeable, and it takes around 60 minutes for caffeine to reach a peak in the blood. This is because caffeine must be absorbed, pass the liver and enter the circulation before it can affect the CNS.

Collagen

Bone, ligaments and tendon and joint health require strong and healthy connective tissue, and all contain collagen as their main protein. Consuming adequate protein is key to maintaining connective tissue health and supplementing with gelatine or hydrolysed collagen with vitamin C can assist with this.

- What is it?
  - » Collagen is a protein your body makes by combining amino acids when you eat protein-rich foods.

- What does it do?
  - » Supplementing with collagen has been shown to help improve connective tissue health, especially after injury.

- Dose:
  - » Take 15 g gelatine or hydrolysed collagen with 50 mg of vitamin C 40–60 minutes prior to exercise, training, rehab, etc.

- What type?
  - » You can buy collagen and vitamin C powder or shots.

Protein Powder

- What is it?
  - » Protein powders are powdered forms of protein from specific sources.

- What does it do?
  - » Protein from powders will work the same way as protein from foods. Although they are not necessarily required in the diet, protein powders can be a safe, efficient way to increase your protein intake. This is especially helpful for individuals aiming for a high protein intake who struggle to get enough from food. Plant-based protein powders can also be helpful for vegetarian or vegan individuals targeting high protein amounts.

- Dose:
  - » One scoop of powder is equal to about 25 g of protein (this can vary depending on the source and scoop size). I do not recommend depending on powders for most of your protein intake. Think of them as a fall-back option of you haven't hit your protein intake by the end of the day.

- What type?
  - » The most common types are whey and casein. These are milk proteins that are both absorbable and effective. There are plant-based protein powders as well, including pea, rice and hemp. However, these protein powders are not as effective as animal-based ones.

Tart Cherry Juice

- What is it?
  - » Tart cherry juice, also known as sour, dwarf or Montmorency cherries, is made from the fruit of the *Prunus cerasus* tree. It is linked to several exercise recovery benefits as it contains many nutrients and beneficial plant compounds.

- What does it do?
  - » It has been shown to accelerate recovery of muscle strength and power, reduce the severity of delayed onset muscle soreness (DOMS) and reduce inflammatory markers. It is also rich in micronutrients so may help immune function and overall health.

- Dose:
  - » Taking 200 mL in the days leading up to and immediately following intense physical exercise may reduce muscle strength soreness and assist with recovery.

- What type?
  - » Look for 'Tart Cherry Juice' or 'Montmorency Cherry Juice'.

Part II

Sleep, Menstrual Cycle and Relative Energy Deficiency in Sport

There are other topics outside of nutrition that I educate my players on. These include sleep, the menstrual cycle, and relative energy deficiency in sport. It is important that you know and understand what effects they may have on your health and performance and how best to manage them. Understanding your own body and needs is the best way to get the most out of it.

Chapter 4

Sleep for Health and Performance

Sleep is a major influencer on your health and performance. It has a significant impact on physical development, cognitive performance, mood and wellbeing. How long and how well you sleep after intense exercise can determine your recovery and training adaptations. Many players that I have worked with over the years were never aware of this, and rarely prioritised their sleep to recover after training and prepare for competition. Do you?

Age	Recommended sleeping hours per 24 hours
3–5 years	10–13 hours
6–12 years	9–12 hours
13–18 year	8–10 hours
18–60 years	7 or more hours
61–64 years	7–9 hours
65 years and older	7–8 hours

Research shows that adequate sleep has a positive effect on reaction times, accuracy, speed and agility (Schwartz et al., 2015). If you are sleep deprived, you may notice your performance or concentration drop. Irritability or low mood due to lack of sleep may affect relationships with your teammates or coaches. Prolonged poor sleep will increase your risk of injury (less than 8 hours sleep has been shown to more than double the risk of injury) and illness (less than 7 hours has been shown to more than triple your risk of illness).

If you find you are experiencing some of the following, it may be a sign that you need more sleep:

- Lack of concentration throughout the day.
- Feeling drowsy during the day.
- Difficulty paying attention.
- Irritability and mood swings.
- Easily falling asleep within 5 minutes of sitting down during the day.
- Frequent illness.
- Frequent injury.

As well as playing a part in how well you recover after training sessions and matches, along with training adaptation, research has shown that if you proactively increase sleep duration and quality it can even improve performance (Mah et al., 2011; Schwartz et al., 2015). Despite the positive effects of sleep on health and performance, players often fail to meet sleep requirements, putting themselves at risk of inadequate recovery, poor performance, illness and injury. There are many obstacles that an athlete might face, including work and study demands, poor sleep environment, stress, training and family responsibilities. Many players will follow an ad hoc schedule when it comes to sleep and, by doing so, may overlook this significant element of their health and performance.

Here are some suggestions on how to improve sleep. They are a mix of evidence-based recommendations and some anecdotal suggestions. Sleep is very subjective, and I like to think of it as something that you need to actively work on. You should work proactively to improve your sleep duration and quality. Much like trying to improve your speed by sprinting or your strength with resistance exercise, sleep improvement should become part of your training schedule!

Tips to improve sleep:

- Avoid alcohol
  - » Alcohol interrupts sleep, it alters melatonin production and results in a poorer quality sleep.

- Reduce caffeine
  - » Even moderate caffeine consumption 6 hours before bed can disrupt sleep. If you rely on a cup of coffee to get you through the afternoon but, in turn, it disrupts your sleep, you need to reduce your caffeine intake.

- Shower or bath
  - » This has been shown to help individuals fall asleep faster – try having a hot bath or shower about 90 minutes before bed.

- Weighted blanket
  - » Sleeping with a weighted blanked may improve sleep duration and quality.

- Routine
  - » Build a positive sleep routine. Go to bed and wake up the same time every day. Your body will then anticipate when it is due to go to sleep, and you will spend less time tossing and turning in bed at night.

- Quality sleep environment
  - » You will spend about a third of your life sleeping. Invest in a decent mattress, appropriate duvet and comfortable pillows. We sleep best in a cool, dark, quiet environment. Use black-out blinds, an eye mask or earplugs if required.

Following a 'sleep timeline' can help as well. Try the following if you are struggling to fall asleep at night:

- Eight hours before bed: avoid caffeine.
- Two hours before bed: Avoid large meals, switch from overhead lights to side lamps, reduce screen time.
- Thirty minutes before bed: get into bed, avoid all screens, read a book with dimmed lighting.
- Five minutes before bed: sleep time, ensure your room is dark, quiet and cool.

Chapter 5

The Menstrual Cycle

Throughout the month, your menstrual cycle may impact your performance due to fluctuating hormones. These fluctuating hormones affect not only your performance but your mood, your energy levels, your recovery and your food choices.

Research has shown that most female athletes have never discussed their menstrual cycle with their coaches and have never received any education about how it relates to their athletic performance (Brown et al., 2021). Given that a lot of team coaches and managers are male, many female players may feel awkward discussing their period with them. Thankfully, this is something that is changing in both elite and recreational sports, but we must keep working to improve the education and communication around this topic. Considering nearly all young female players will have a period, there's a high probability that during any given team training session or game, at least some of the players will be menstruating. Thus, periods and the impact they can have on players, both positive and negative, is something that should be understood and considered by athletes and their coaches.

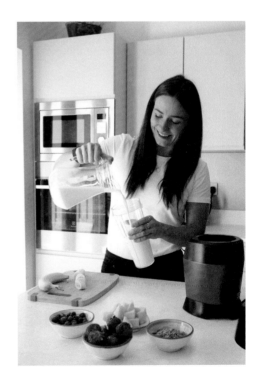

Let's start by breaking down the four phases in the menstrual cycle:

1. Menstruation (Day 1–5)

Menstruation is when the thickened lining of the womb (uterus) sheds through the vagina. This lining fluid contains blood, cells and mucus. Although it can vary, the average length of a period is between 3 and 7 days.

2. Follicular phase (Day 1–13)

The follicular phase starts on the first day of menstruation and ends with ovulation. Prompted by the hypothalamus, the pituitary gland releases follicle stimulating hormone. During this phase, the hormone oestrogen will also start to rise due to the developing follicle.

3. Ovulation (Day 14)

Ovulation is the release of a mature egg from the surface of the ovary. This usually occurs mid-cycle, around two weeks before menstruation starts. Oestrogen peaks just before ovulation, and then drops shortly afterwards.

4. Luteal phase (Day 15–28)

This phase refers to the time between ovulation and the start of menstruation when the body prepares for a possible pregnancy. Progesterone is produced, along with a small amount of oestrogen. Both hormones rise and then drop. These hormonal changes are associated with common premenstrual symptoms (PMS) that many women experience.

— Oestrogen
— Progesterone

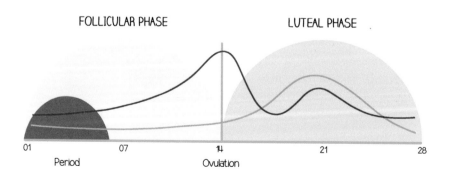

FOLLICULAR PHASE   LUTEAL PHASE

01   07   14   21   28
Period   Ovulation

If pregnancy does not occur, the drop in progesterone levels causes the lining of the womb to fall away as the cycle begins again and you get your period. Like many things in life, not all periods are clockwork or exactly as described above. Many players think they experience irregular cycles (oligomenorrhoea); however, you can be outside the 28-day cycle and still considered regular. Any cycle between 21 and 35 days is classed as 'normal' (and even up to 40 days in adolescent girls). It is also normal for your own cycle to vary month to month, for example it can be 26 days one month and 30 the next! If a woman regularly goes more than 35 days without menstruating, or has only 4–9 cycles a year, then it is termed as oligomenorrhoea.

How the Menstrual Cycle Affects Performance

Due to the rise and fall of your hormones, you may experience some impact on your performance throughout the month. The effect your cycle has on performance will vary from person to person. Some athletes will be more sensitive to hormonal changes than others, and this sensitivity may also change as you get older. Even though excellent research has been carried out in recent years, and very exciting studies are ongoing in this area, there is still no conclusive guidance about how your performance is going to be influenced throughout the month. However, from what we do know, there are some things you can expect as you move through the phases of your cycle:

Follicular phase

When you get your period – and in the early follicular phase – hormones are at their lowest; this may mean additional energy is available that can be used for exercise. Many women report that they feel strongest during this time and often hit exercise personal bests! As you move into the late follicular phase and approach ovulation, tolerance to higher-intensity training may reduce.

Luteal phase

Following ovulation, your hormones will start to rise, and your body may have a harder time recovering from high-intensity workouts. As you move into the late luteal phase, you become premenstrual and dramatic hormone changes may make it harder for your body to perform optimally.

Tracking Your Period

Tracking your menstrual cycle is incredibly beneficial. It can help you identify any changes in your performance and training across your cycle. In turn, this can then help you to either enhance or reduce these effects. Aside from performance benefits, when you track your cycle, you will know when to expect your period (and plan for it accordingly), notice any changes or irregularities and you will be able to reduce/increase the chance of pregnancy. There are numerous tracking apps you can download and use, including ones that are specifically for athletes. If you want a simpler approach, you can use the notes section or calendar on your phone or even a good old pen and paper! I would recommend tracking in as much detail as you can when you start. Start the first day of your period and track any symptoms you experience (type of flow, cramps, energy levels, mood, sleep, etc.). Continue for the rest of the month. Make note of how your training feels throughout the month and any other changes in performance or mood. Track for at least 3 months and then review. Make note of any obvious patterns – do you feel energised the week of your period? Did you feel training got harder around the time of ovulation? Did you struggle to fuel up after you got your period due to cramps or lack of appetite? Use this information to make any appropriate adjustments to your training and nutrition. The better your understanding of your cycle's impact on your own performance, the better you will be able to prepare and adapt to these changes.

The Hormonal Contraceptive (HC)

When you are on an HC, your oestrogen and progesterone production is suppressed, which results in a steady hormonal profile throughout the month. This leads us to believe that there should be little differences in performance throughout your monthly cycle. However, some women might be very susceptible to even minute hormonal changes, which could then affect training, mood, recovery and/or performance. I would still recommend tracking if you are on an HC, as this will help you understand how it affects different areas of your physiology and mood. This, in turn, will help you understand what influences it has on your performance and exercise. As nearly all apps are designed for those who are tracking a natural menstrual cycle, it might be best to use an excel file or notebook to track your HC cycle. Track for a minimum of 3 months and assess your notes every 4 weeks. Look for patterns that seem to affect your training, energy levels and/or mood, then make appropriate adjustments to improve these areas. There are lots of things to make note of, but I would recommend including the following:

- Emotional changes day to day.
- Energy levels.
- Withdrawal bleeds (start and end date, blood flow amount).
- Physical changes.
- Weekly performance assessment.

Relative Energy Deficiency in Sport

Relative Energy Deficiency in Sport (RED-S) is a condition among athletes caused by low energy availability (LEA). LEA arises when caloric intake doesn't meet the requirements for bodily function and exercise. RED-S is a condition that describes the consequences of prolonged LEA on bodily processes, including menstrual function, cardiovascular function, gastrointestinal health, bone health, growth and development, and overall health and wellbeing. It impairs performance and affects both female and male athletes of all ages and levels who do not fuel adequately. This inadequate fuelling can be either intentional or unintentional.

Avoiding LEA can be challenging for female athletes. It is relatively common among young women participating in sport and arises when energy intake is insufficient to cover the combined energy (calorie) demands of training and baseline physiological processes to maintain health. The body responds to this insufficient energy intake by switching off 'nonessential' bodily processes (menstrual cycle) to keep other biological systems functioning optimally (cardiovascular, immune, etc.).

When we don't eat enough to meet our energy demands (or over exercise), the first thing that is usually affected is our menstrual function. It may lighten, become irregular (oligomenorrhoea) or stop completely (amenorrhoea). If you notice changes in your period, it may be a sign that your body is under stress, therefore, it is essential that, as an athlete, you track your period.

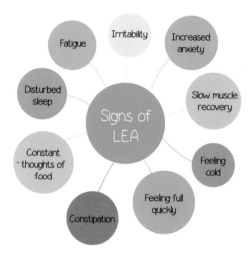

As well your menstrual cycle, there are other signs to be aware of. You should keep RED-S in mind if you have noticed any changes in your health and/or performance. Please see the following graphic for the RED-S clinical assessment tool (RED-S CAT). This is used to detect red flags for LEA and RED-S in athletes. If you are experiencing any of the symptoms, please speak with a medical professional. If these warning signings go unaddressed, the symptoms will worsen, and you may place yourself at risk of irreparable damage to your body. Be mindful of any increased training load. This can be in the form of additional, longer duration or higher-intensity training sessions. As your training load goes up, so should your energy intake. This to ensure you do not place yourself at risk of LEA.

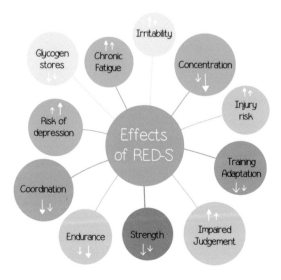

○ Do I feel tired all the time even when getting adequate sleep?

○ Am I excessively sore and feeling like I can't quite recover between sessions?

○ Is my performance failing to improve at the rate my coaches are expecting?

○ Is my mood low or fluctuating?

○ Have I had reoccurring injuries in the last year?

○ Have I ever had a stress fracture?

○ Am I frequently ill or sick?

○ Is my menstrual cycle irregular, lighter than normal, or absent?

Part III

Recipes

We are now into the practical side of this book. Knowing what you should eat to fuel and recover from training and matches is all well and good, but it is of little benefit unless you do it! Here you will learn:

- What kitchen essentials you need to follow my recipes
- How to meal prep
- How to cook commonly eaten foods
- When and why to choose certain recipes
- How to plan your training and match weeks

Chapter 6

Cooking

Kitchen Essentials

If you are trying to master some healthy recipes, make sure your kitchen has the essentials. Many out there are overwhelmed by the thoughts of meal prep and healthy cooking. Remove barriers by setting up your kitchen with the basic tools you need to try new recipes.

Here I have listed some essential cooking tools to help you follow most recipes. If you have a few missing from your kitchen, make it a priority to get one thing you need a week – most can be found in your local supermarket. Having these basic tools will help your confidence with cooking and trying new recipes!

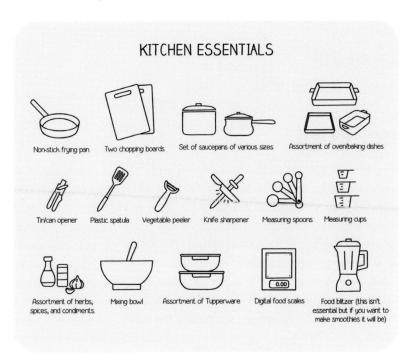

KITCHEN ESSENTIALS

Non-stick frying pan   Two chopping boards   Set of saucepans of various sizes   Assortment of oven/baking dishes

Tin/can opener   Plastic spatula   Vegetable peeler   Knife sharpener   Measuring spoons   Measuring cups

Assortment of herbs, spices, and condiments.   Mixing bowl   Assortment of Tupperware   Digital food scales   Food blitzer (this isn't essential but if you want to make smoothies it will be)

I was a college student when my love for cooking first started. I started out with relatively easy recipes, however, the biggest roadblock I faced was my lack of seasonings! A stocked seasoning cupboard will make for easy cooking and tasty dishes. You don't need to go and buy everything at once, but just pick up one or two things every time you're in the supermarket. It won't be long until you have everything you could possibly need to make a delicious meal on short notice.

Spice (dried)	Herb	Condiments/oils
Black pepper	Basil	Extra Virgin Olive oil
Paprika	Oregano	Vinegar
Cumin	Parsley	Hot sauce
Cayenne	Chives	Sesame oil
Turmeric	Dill	Coconut oil
Curry powder	Thyme	Honey
Chilli Powder	Rosemary	Stock cubes
Chilli flakes	Sage	Salt
Fajita seasoning	Mixed herbs	
Ginger		
Cinnamon		
Coriander (Cilantro)		

Meal Prep

Prepping some of your meals for the week can really help when you are trying to make positive habit changes. That's not to say that you must spend your Sundays doing multiple batch cooks or anything, but making enough for two or three portions when you are preparing a meal might take a little longer but will save you a lot of time and effort in the following days. This is why you will see some of my recipes will make multiple portions. Imagine you have had a long day at work, you then have training and, by the time you are home, the last thing you want to do is try to cook a meal from scratch. This is a habit that will not only save you time and money but will also ensure you are making the right choices when it comes to your health and performance. Surplus meals can be stored in the fridge for a couple of days, or if you want to be really prepared, you can keep a cache of training and recovery day meals in Tupperware in your freezer.

Cooking 101

If you bought this book because you finally want to take control of your nutrition and start preparing your own meals, then this next section is for you. A lot of people have never been shown how to cook growing up. I was brought up on a typical Irish country diet (mostly meat, potatoes and two veg meals). There was nothing wrong with this (thanks, Mam!); however, it did mean that I found it daunting to try recipes from different cuisines or more complex dishes. Understanding the basics can go a long way when you are deciding if you want to try new recipes. Here are some of the fundamentals to help you.

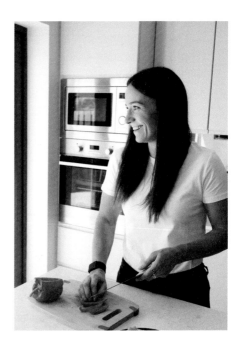

Prepping Vegetables

If there's one thing that's going to make veg prep hard, it's blunt knives! Make sure you take 30 seconds sharpening your knives before you start peeling and chopping your vegetables!

Measuring Ingredients

I recommend that you have digital food scales, measuring cups and measuring spoons in your kitchen. These aren't expensive and will ensure you can follow any recipes you might like to try. Digital food scales are great; you simply place a bowl or pot on the scale, set it to zero and then add your ingredient. My recipes are in grams, millilitres, tablespoons or teaspoons. Some foods (mostly fruit and vegetables) will be less specific and will just ask for a 'medium carrot', or 'half a head of broccoli'.

How to Cook Pasta

1. Boil the kettle – this will help speed up your cooking time as you won't have to wait for water to boil in a pan.
2. Fill a large saucepan with the boiled water, place the lid on and bring to the boil over a high heat.
3. Add a couple of pinches of salt.
4. When the water starts to boil, add the pasta, stir occasionally so it doesn't stick.
5. Cook the pasta according to the packet instructions. Before the packet cooking time is over, try a piece to see if it is cooked. It's ready when it's soft enough to eat, but still has a bit of bite. You don't want to overcook it as it can go mushy.
6. As a rule, I always scoop out a mugful of the starchy cooking water. This will help thicken a pasta sauce if required.
7. Drain the pasta in a colander over the sink.

How to Cook Rice

1. Measure out the rice according to the recipe and rinse thoroughly with cold water until it runs clear. If time allows, soak the rice in cold water for at least 30 minutes (this help it cook evenly but isn't compulsory).
2. Pour the rice into a pan over a low heat, then add the butter or oil, if using, and stir to coat the rice grains.
3. Boil the kettle, this will help speed up your cooking time as you won't have to wait for water to boil in a pan.
4. Add double the amount of water (e.g. 200 mL water for a 100 g serving).
5. Bring to a boil and stir once to make sure the rice is evenly distributed.
6. Put a lid on and turn the heat down to low. If you cook the rice on too high a heat, it will cook too quickly and may end up dry and flaky in the centre.
7. Cook for about 10 minutes with the lid on all the time. Then check the rice is cooked by trying a small spoonful.
8. Fluff the rice with a fork and serve!

How to Tell if a Potato is Cooked?

The length of time a potato takes to cook depends on its size. So, if you're making mashed potatoes, it's worth taking a couple of minutes to chop your potatoes into small cubes. To tell if the potato is cooked, pierce with a fork. If the fork goes through with little resistance, then your spud is cooked!

How to Tell if Chicken/Turkey is Cooked?

It is vital that you cook poultry fully before you eat it. To ensure that your meat is safely cooked check for the following signs:

1. That the meat is steaming hot all the way through.
2. Cut into the thickest part of the meal and ensure that there is no pink meat visible.
3. The juices should run clear when you pierce the meat.

How to Tell if Fish is Cooked?

Although most fish can be eaten raw (think of sushi), most of us prefer that it is cooked when including it in our meals! To tell if fish is cooked, test it with a fork at the thickest point. Insert the fork at an angle and twist gently. The fish will flake easily when it's done and won't be translucent or raw in appearance.

Eggs

Eggs are one of my favourite foods, so much so that I even have hens in my back garden that provide fresh eggs for my breakfast every morning! Eggs are suited to every meal and are one of the most versatile foods for cooking. They are high in protein and are absolutely packed with vitamins and minerals. So, to use these little nutrient bombs we should be able to cook them properly! I've outlined the main four ways to cook eggs so that you can follow any recipe that includes them.

Fried

A good non-stick pan is essential when tackling new recipes and, when it comes to things like fried eggs, it can help make some tasty meals! If your egg gets stuck to the pan, it will break and you'll have to settle for some scrambled eggs! For the perfect fried egg, follow these steps:

* To ensure you don't end up with eggshells in your pan, crack the egg onto a small saucer. Slide it off the saucer into the pan.
* Cover with a lid and then leave for about 3 minutes over a low heat. Check the white is set. If the egg white is still running, place the lid back on, leave it for another 30 seconds and check again. If you prefer your egg yolk set, you can flip the egg with a plastic spatula. Season with salt and pepper.

Scrambled

If you have never cooked eggs before, scrambled eggs are the ones to start with as it's fairly hard to go wrong with them!

* Whisk eggs, half a teaspoon of butter, salt and pepper in a small bowl.
* Place your non-stick frying pan over medium-high heat.
* Pour in egg mixture and reduce heat to medium-low.
* As eggs begin to set, gently move them with a plastic or rubber spatula around the pan to form large, soft curds.
* Keep moving the eggs until they have thickened but no liquid egg remains but be sure not to overcook the eggs as they will dry quite quickly.

Boiled

I love the simplicity of boiled eggs – no mess, no fuss, all the taste! To cook them you simply boil them in a small saucepan for as long as you wish, depending on how you like them cooked.

* Five minutes: egg white just set and very runny yolk.
* Six minutes: egg white set and liquid yolk.
* Seven minutes: egg white set and yolk sticky, almost set.
* Eight minutes: egg white set and yolk softly set.
* Ten minutes: egg white set and yolk set.

Poached

Poached eggs can be daunting at first, but I promise, after a bit of practice, you will be topping your brunch recipes with some perfectly cooked poached eggs!

* Fill a pan with at least 2 inches of water, bring it to a rolling boil (just above a simmer). Add a teaspoon of vinegar.
* Crack your egg into a cup.
* With a large spoon, stir the water to create a gentle whirlpool. This will help the egg white wrap around the yolk.
* Slowly tip the egg out of the cup into the centre of the whirlpool. Cook for 3–4 minutes or until the white is set.
* Use a large, slotted spoon to lift the egg out onto some kitchen paper.

Chapter 7

How to Choose Your Recipes

Some of you reading this book will have never cooked before, and some will be experienced in the kitchen and confident in your abilities. Taking that into consideration, I have created these recipes so that they not only taste great but are also easy to follow and accessible to all. I recommend that before you choose a recipe, read through it first and get familiar with it. I have included the length of time the recipe takes to cook; however, a longer recipe does not necessarily mean that it is harder to cook, but it may have more components to prepare.

My recipes have been created, tried, tested, adjusted and perfected over many years. I hope you enjoy them as much as I, my family, friends and followers in social media have. There are a mix of meat, fish, vegetarian and vegan dishes. If you follow a meat-free diet, you can substitute the meat for a plant-based alternative; please note that this will change the nutrient profile provided with the recipe.

The recipes are broken up into two categories:

1. Training days
2. Recovery days

The training day recipes are suited to days of moderate-to-high intensity training, the day before a game or game days. They have a higher carbohydrate, moderate protein and lower fat content. As previously discussed in chapter 3, this is the recommended macronutrient ratio for fuelling meals. Using these recipes as your main meals and incorporating high carb snacks will ensure you are fuelling correctly on training and match days.

Recovery day recipes are designed to ensure you are meeting your required nutrients for recovery and health. They are higher in fibre, healthy fats, protein and have more vegetables than the training day recipes. These nutrient-dense meals will boost your essential nutrient intake and enable you to recover adequately between training sessions and matches. These recipes are also ideal for off season or if you are out of training with an injury. Obviously, you are free to mix and match these recipes as you see fit. Use the sample training and recovery day meal plans as a guide for how to plan your week. I have also combined them all to show how it might fit together for a week of training. There is also a Game Week sample plan.

You can modify the recipes as well if you prefer. If you like the look of a training day recipe but don't have any exercise planned, you can decrease the carbohydrate and increase the protein, vegetables and/or fat. Similarly, to modify a recovery meal to a training one, increase the carb source and decrease the protein, vegetables and/or fat. I'd recommend following the recipes as they are first. This will give you a good idea of what high carbohydrate meals look like. You can then try to replicate them by modifying recovery day recipes as this will ensure you are adequately fuelling.

To help get you started, make a few lists, such as the first five training day recipes you want to try or the first five recovery day recipes you want to try. That way you can easily plan your week and your shopping trips.

Training Week Sample Meal Plan (yellow for medium carb, green for high carb)

	Monday (6 a.m. gym session)	Tuesday (7 p.m. pitch/ court training)	Wednesday (recovery day)	Thursday (7 p.m. pitch/ court training)	Friday (6 p.m. gym session)	Saturday (recovery day)	Sunday (10 a.m. pitch/ court training)
Pre-gym/ training snack	Banana and coffee	***	***	***	***	***	Small bowl of rice cereal and coffee
Recovery snack	500 mL low-fat milk	***	***	***	***	***	500 mL low-fat milk and a banana
Breakfast	Chickpea and Avo Toast	Loaded Porridge and large glass of OJ	Rushing Around Breakfast Baked Bar and a banana	Loaded Porridge large glass of OJ	Smoothie Bowl	Breakfast Burrito	Chocolate Protein Pancake Stack
Mid-morning snack	Apple slices and peanut butter	Dried apricots and almonds	Mixed nuts and large bunch of grapes	Oatcakes, almond butter, large orange	Mixed nuts and large bunch of grapes	Apple slices and peanut butter	Dried apricots and almonds
Lunch	Prawn and Mango Salad	Folded Chicken Wraps	Peri Peri Chicken Pitta	Beetroot and Couscous Wrap	Cheesy Stuffed Peppers	Mexican Quinoa	Easy Veegy Baked Beans
Mid-afternoon snack	Yogurt, pumpkin seeds, pear	Pineapple Fuel Smoothie	Yogurt, pumpkin seeds, pear	Granola Bar and an apple	BN PB Protein Bars	Protein Peanut Butter Cups and a pear	Granola bar and an apple
Pre-training snack	****	Granola and yogurt	***	Berry Fuel Smoothie	Banana	***	***
Post-training snack	****	Strawberry Choc Smoothie	***	500 mL milk, Recovery Bar, banana	500 mL low-fat milk	***	***
Dinner	Beef Chow Mein	Chicken Fajita Pasta	Pan-Fried Salmon and Sweet Potato	Prawn and Coconut Thai Curry	All the Spuds Fish Pie	Prawn & Chorizo Jam-balaya	Tomato Pasta Bake
Pre-bed snack	Yogurt, chia seeds, mixed berries	***	Wholegrain toast, peanut butter, glass of milk	***	Overnight Muscle Builder smoothie	Wheety Banana Breakfast	Yogurt, chia seeds, mixed berries

Game Week Sample Meal Plan (yellow for medium carb, green for high carb)

	Monday (6 a.m. gym session)	Tuesday (7 p.m. pitch/ court training)	Wednesday (recovery day)	Thursday (7 p.m. pitch/ court training)	Friday (Game day -1)	Saturday (5 p.m. game)	Sunday (Recovery day)
Pre-gym/ training snack	Banana and coffee	***	***	***	***	***	***
Recovery snack	500 mL low-fat milk	***	***	***	***	***	***
Breakfast	Egg Galette	Blue Cash on Toasted Sourdough and a large glass of apple juice	Veggie Breakfast	PB & A Porridge and a large glass of apple juice	Smoothie Bowl	On-The-Go Overnight Oats and a large glass of OJ	French Toast
Mid-morning snack	Mixed nuts and large bunch of grapes	Dried apricots and almonds	Mixed nuts and large bunch of grapes	Oatcakes, almond butter, large orange	Mixed nuts and large bunch of grapes	Giddy Up Granola and Yogurt	Crispy Quinoa Bar, apple
Lunch	Chicken Fajita Salad	Easy Veegy Baked Beans	Sticky Beef and Asparagus	Sweet Potato Toast and Hummus	Mexican Chicken and Quinoa	Sun-dried Tomato Pesto Pasta	Quick Que-sadillas
Mid-afternoon snack	Egg Cups, apple	Two slices of toast with sliced banana and honey	Yogurt, pumpkin seeds, pear	Fuelling Flapjack and an apple	Cream crackers with cheese, large orange	Crumpets with jam, apple, granola bar	Yogurt, chia seeds, mixed berries
Pre-training/ match snack	****	Fuelling Flapjack	***	Berry Fuel Smoothie	***	Berry Fuel Smoothie, cereal bar, jellies	***
Post-training/ match snack	****	Choc Malt Shake	***	500 mL milk, Crispy Quinoa Bar, banana	***	Fruitie Smoothie	***
Dinner	Pesto Salmon & Roast Veg	Taco Mince and Rice	Mexican Lasagne	Spiced Carrot and Lentil Soup	Basil Pesto Spaghetti	Chilli Con Carne	Seafood Tagliatelle
Pre-bed snack	Yogurt, chia seeds, mixed berries	***	Egg Cups	***	Wheety Banana Breakfast	***	High Protein Brownie, glass of milk

Chapter 8

Training Day Recipes

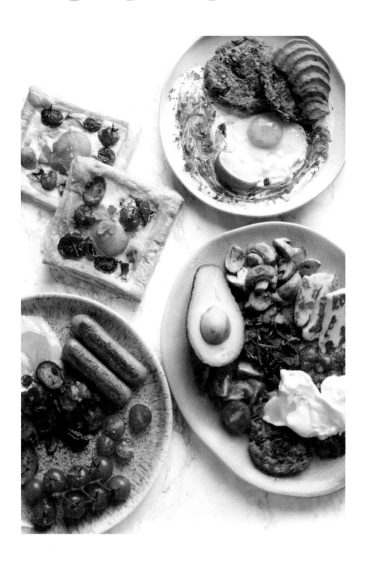

Training Day Breakfasts

Chocolate Protein Pancake Stack

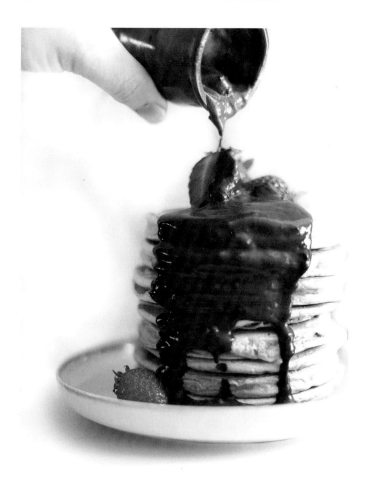

These are a firm favourite in my house. Great for when you have a little more time at the weekend to prepare a nice breakfast.

Servings: 2

Time to make: 30 minutes

Vegetarian

Ingredients

* 60 g porridge (oatmeal)
* 3 eggs
* 1 banana
* 1 scoop of protein powder chocolate/vanilla
* 1 teaspoon of coconut oil
* 1 protein bar (chocolate-based one)
* 3–4 tablespoons of milk
* Handful of strawberries, halved
* 10 hazelnuts, chopped

Instructions

1. Blitz the porridge until you have a coarse flour.
2. Add the eggs, banana, and protein powder.
3. Heat the oil in a large non-stick pan over medium to high heat.
4. Add 3–4 tablespoons of batter to the pan to make a medium pancake.
5. Cook for 1–2 minutes on each side, until it is browned.
6. Make 8 pancakes.
7. While the pancakes are cooking, break up the bar and heat for 20 seconds in the microwave.
8. Add a tablespoon of milk and stir.
9. Heat the bar again for 20 seconds and keep stirring. The chocolate will easily burn so be careful.
10. Add the remaining milk and stir until you have a sauce like consistency.
11. Stack the pancakes and strawberries as shown in the picture on two plates.
12. Pour over the sauce and top each stack with the hazelnuts.
13. Devour.

Nutrient Info Per Serving

Calories: 542 | Carbs: 39 g | Fibre: 12 g | Protein: 40 g | Fat: 20 g | Saturated Fat: 6.7 g

Loaded Porridge

Oats are an athlete's best friend. They are an excellent slow-releasing carb source and are one of the most versatile foods out there!

Servings: 1

Time to make: 5 minutes

Vegetarian

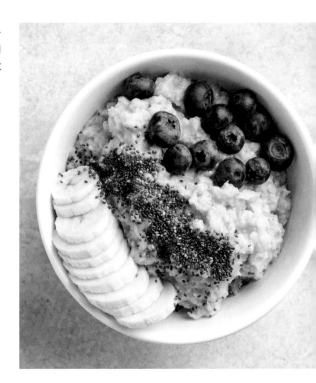

Ingredients
- 70 g porridge oats (oatmeal)
- 250 mL of milk
- Pinch of salt
- 1 teaspoon of chia seeds
- 1 teaspoon of flaxseeds
- 1 handful of blueberries
- 1 chopped banana
- 1 tablespoon of honey

Instructions
1. Add oats to a small saucepan, pour in milk and sprinkle in a pinch of salt. Bring to the boil and simmer for 4–5 minutes, stirring from time to time and watching carefully that it doesn't stick to the bottom of the pan.
2. Or you can try this in a microwave. Mix the porridge oats, milk, and a pinch of salt in a bowl, then microwave on high for 3–4 minutes, stirring halfway through.
3. To serve, pour into a bowl, top with chia seeds, flaxseeds, blueberries, chopped banana and honey.

Nutrient Info Per Serving
Calories: 501 | Carbs: 77 g | Fibre: 8 g | Protein: 20 g | Fa: 11 g | Saturated Fat: 2.6 g

Wheety Banana Breakfast

Another quick training day breakfast! Adding fruit to your fuelling breakfast will help bump up the carbs and get you ready for the day ahead.

Servings: 1

Time to make: 5 minutes

Vegetarian

Ingredients
- 3 wheat biscuits
- 1 banana, chopped
- 1 tablespoon of honey
- 300 mL of milk

Instructions
1. Combine all ingredients in a bowl.
2. Enjoy the fuelling breakfast hot or cold!

Nutrient Info Per Serving
Calories: 500 | Carbs: 92 g | Fibre: 7 g | Protein: 20 g | Fat: 4 g | Saturated Fat: 2 g

French Toast

This is one of my favourite training day options. Slightly stale bread works best. Get inventive with the toppings!

Servings: 1

Time to make: 15 minutes

Vegetarian

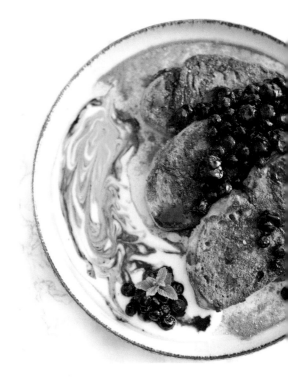

Ingredients
* 1 egg
* 30 mL milk
* Pinch of salt
* Half a teaspoon of cinnamon
* 1 teaspoon of butter
* 2 slices of wholegrain bread
* 1 handful of blueberries
* 1 tablespoon of honey
* 150 g natural yogurt

Instructions
1. Add the eggs, milk, salt and cinnamon to a bowl and whisk.
2. Heat the butter over a medium heat.
3. Soak the bread in the egg mix and fry until golden brown on both sides, about 3–4 minutes.
4. Add the blueberries and honey to a saucepan, bring to the boil, reduce the heat and simmer for a couple of minutes.
5. Serve the toast with yogurt and the berry compote.

Nutrient Info Per Serving
Calories: 539 | Carbs: 65 g | Fibre: 5 g | Protein: 24 g | Fat: 19 g | Saturated Fat: 9.5 g

PB & A Porridge

The classic flavour combination of apple and peanut butter added to oats to make a delicious fuelling porridge.

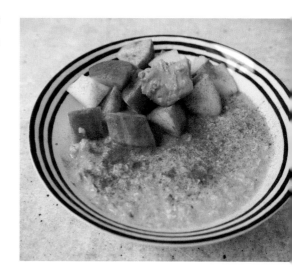

Servings: 1

Time to make: 5 minutes

Vegetarian

Ingredients

- 1 apple, chopped
- 80 g porridge oats (oatmeal)
- 250 mL of milk
- Pinch of salt
- 1 heaped teaspoon of peanut butter
- 1 tablespoon of honey
- Half a teaspoon of cinnamon

Instructions

1. Chop the apple and add to a bowl. Microwave for 1–2 minutes until just tender. Make sure to use a large bowl so the porridge doesn't bubble over when cooked.
2. Put the oats, milk and a pinch of salt in the bowl, then microwave on high for 3–4 minutes, stirring halfway through.
3. To serve, pour into bowls, top with the peanut butter, honey and cinnamon.

Nutrient Info Per Serving

Calories: 689 | Carbs: 109 g | Fibre: 10 g | Protein: 24 g | Fat: 17 g | Saturated Fat: 4.5 g

Giddy Up Granola and Yogurt

I make this at the start of the week and use it for training days as a breakfast option or in snacks!

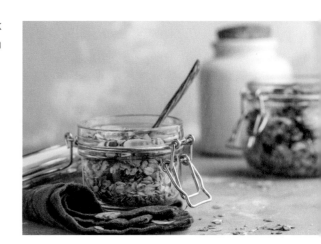

Servings: 3

Time to make: 30 minutes

Vegan

Ingredients

- 1 teaspoon of coconut oil
- 2 tablespoons of honey
- 1 teaspoon of vanilla extract
- 150 g porridge oats (oatmeal)
- 30 g plain cashew nuts
- 2 tablespoons of pumpkin seeds
- 2 tablespoons of sesame seeds
- 50 g dried cranberries
- 50 g dried blueberries
- 2 tablespoons of natural yogurt with each serving

Instructions

1. Heat oven to 150°C / fan 130°C / 300°F / gas mark 2.
2. Melt the coconut oil in a large bowl in the microwave for 30 seconds.
3. Add the honey and vanilla and mix well.
4. Tip in all the remaining ingredients, except the dried fruit, and mix well.
5. Tip the granola onto two baking sheets and spread evenly.
6. Bake for 15 minutes, then mix in the dried fruit, and bake for 10–15 minutes more.
7. Remove and scrape onto a flat tray to cool.
8. Serve with 2 tablespoons of yogurt.
9. The granola can be stored in an airtight container for up to a month.

Nutrient Info Per Serving (with yogurt)

Calories: 560 | **Carbs:** 70 g | **Fibre:** 8 g | **Protein:** 18 g | **Fat:** 22 g | **Saturated Fat:** 7 g

On-the-Go Overnight Oats

A great option for those who like to be prepared on training days! Make the night before and grab from the fridge as you're heading out the door.

Servings: 1

Time to make: 5 minutes

Vegetarian

Ingredients

- 60 g porridge oats (oatmeal)
- 1 banana chopped
- 2 teaspoons of chia seeds
- 1 tablespoon of honey
- 300 mL milk

Instructions

1. Place all ingredients into a container and mix until combined.
2. Cover the container with a lid or plastic wrap. Place in the fridge overnight.
3. Grab from the fridge the next morning and enjoy on the go. Thin with a little more milk or water, if desired.

Nutrient Info Per Serving

Calories: 558 | Carbs: 91 g | Fibre: 8 g | Protein: 21 g | Fat: 10 g | Saturated Fat: 2.8 g

Breakfast Smoothie

This is for those who don't like to eat a big breakfast, or who might feel too nervous to eat the morning of a game. This fuelling smoothie packs a punch to get you on your way!

Servings: 1

Time to make: 5 minutes

Vegetarian

Ingredients

- 20 g porridge oats (oatmeal)
- 1 apple, chopped
- 1 tablespoon of flaxseed
- 1 tablespoon of chia seeds
- 1 handful of mixed berries
- 400 mL milk
- 1 tablespoon of honey

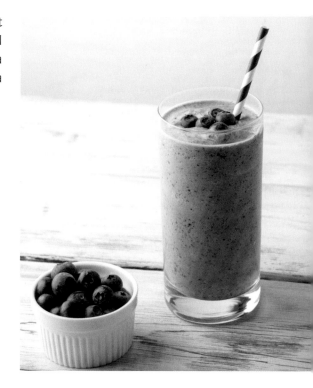

Instructions

1. Add all ingredients to a blender and blitz.
2. Add some water if it is a little thick.

Nutrient Info Per Serving

Calories: 587 | Carbs: 81 g | Fibre: 13 g | Protein: 25 g | Fat: 15 g | Saturated Fat: 3.7 g

Blue Cash on Toasted Sourdough

This is a fancy spin on a PB and J sandwich! Packed with healthy fats and carbs, this is an ideal way to start your fuelling.

Servings: 1

Time to make: 10 minutes

Vegan

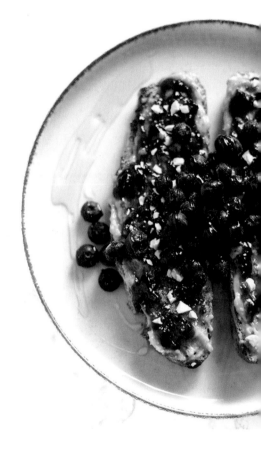

Ingredients

- 2 slices of sourdough
- 1 tablespoon of honey
- 60 g frozen blueberries
- 1 tablespoon of chia seeds
- 2 tablespoons of cashew nut butter
- 5 cashew nuts, chopped

Instructions

1. Toast the sourdough.
2. When the bread is toasting, add the honey, blueberries and seeds to a small pot over a medium heat.
3. Stir until the berries have thawed and the mix bubbles, then remove from the heat.
4. Top the toast with an even amount of nut butter and the berry seed mix.
5. Sprinkle over the chopped cashews.

Nutrient Info Per Serving

Calories: 649 | Carbs: 71 g | Fibre: 14 g | Protein: 20 g | Fat: 29 g | Saturated Fat: 5.4 g

Quick Quinoa Proats

You might think it's odd to have quinoa for breakfast, but I promise you this versatile grain works great for any meal! It is high in protein and an important plant source of all nine EAAs.

Servings: 1

Time to make: 10 minutes

Vegetarian

Ingredients

- 100 g cooked quinoa
- 40 g porridge oats (oatmeal)
- 1 scoop of protein powder (any favour you like)
- 300 mL milk
- 2 tablespoons of dried blueberries
- 1 tablespoon of goji berries
- 1 tablespoon of honey

Instructions

1. Add the cooked quinoa, oats, protein powder and milk to a bowl and leave to soak overnight.
2. When you are ready to eat, top with the berries and honey.
3. Enjoy!

Nutrient Info Per Serving

Calories: 619 | Carbs: 87 g | Fibre: 10 g | Protein: 44 g | Fat: 8 g | Saturated Fat: 1.6 g

Training Day Lunches

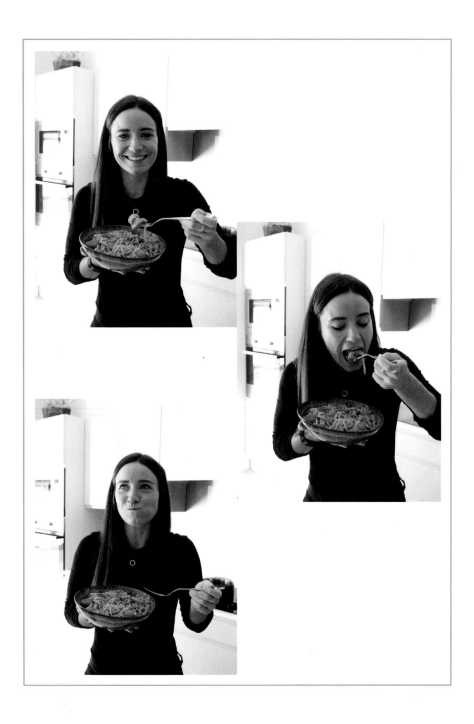

Folded Chicken Wraps

A little twist on your regular wrap. Instead of rolling all the fillings up, the tortilla is folded into quarters, making a compact, triangle-shaped wrap.

Serves: 1

Time to cook: 10 minutes

Ingredients

- 2 tortilla wraps
- 70 g cooked chicken
- 2 handfuls of spinach, chopped
- 1 medium tomato, sliced
- 2 teaspoons of mayo

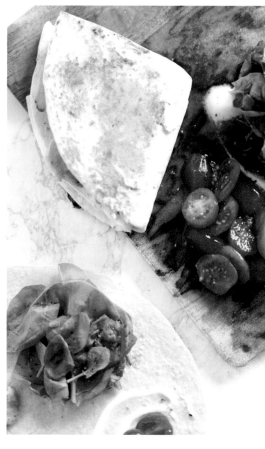

Instructions

1. Lay your tortilla out on a cutting board. Take a knife and make a cut from the centre of the tortilla down to the edge.
2. Imagine the tortilla being divided up into four quarters. Add a different ingredient into each quadrant.
3. Fold the wrap up, starting from the bottom left quarter, folding it up over the top left, then folding it over to the top right, then folding it down to the bottom right. Repeat with the second wrap.
4. Enjoy cold or grill.

Nutrient Info Per Serving

Calories: 631 | Carbs: 65 g | Fibre: 8 g | Protein: 31 g | Fat: 25 g | Saturated Fat: 4 g

Mexican Chicken and Quinoa

Batch cooking high carbohydrate meals at once is an efficient way to ensure you are fuelling well on training days. This is a tasty option, and if you like more heat, you can choose a spicier Chipotle chilli paste.

Serves: 4

Time to cook: 25 minutes

Ingredients

- 1 tablespoon of extra virgin olive oil
- 140 g quinoa (uncooked)
- 1 red onion, chopped
- 300 g chicken, diced
- 1 tablespoon of Chipotle chilli cooking paste
- 1 pepper, chopped
- 1 tin of pinto beans, drained
- 1 tin of tomatoes
- Salt and pepper

Instructions

1. Heat the oil in a large saucepan over a medium heat.
2. Cook the quinoa according to packet instructions in a separate pot of boiling water.
3. When the oil in the saucepan is hot, add the onion and cook for a couple of minutes until soft, then add the chicken and cook for 5 minutes, stirring all the time, season with salt and pepper.
4. Add Chipotle cooking paste, stir through.
5. Add the pepper, beans and tin of tomatoes and stir well.
6. Simmer for 5–7 minutes.
7. Strain the quinoa and add to the pan.
8. Mix well.
9. Divide between 4 dishes/lunch boxes.

Nutrient Info Per Serving

Calories: 487 | Carbs: 56 g | Protein: 35 g | Fat: 10 g | Fibre: 13 g | Saturated Fat: 1.4 g

Fajita Bowl

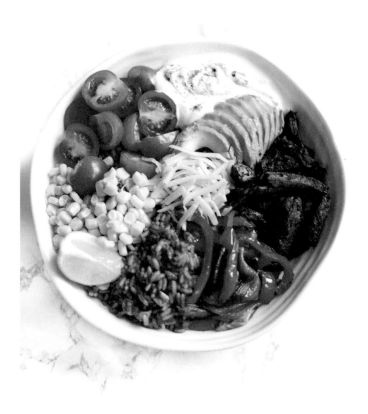

Microwave rice packets are a fuelling hack I've long recommended to athletes. If you prefer to cook the rice, then use 125 g uncooked long grain rice. However, if you're in a hurry (like most of us are), the quick option is perfect for you!

Serves: 2

Time to cook: 30 minutes

Ingredients

- 2 teaspoons of extra virgin olive oil
- 2 small chicken breasts, diced
- 1 pepper, thinly sliced
- Half a red onion, sliced
- 2 teaspoons of fajita seasoning
- Handful of cherry tomatoes, chopped
- 1 lime, cut into quarters
- 1 clove of garlic, finely chopped/crushed
- Half an avocado, mashed
- 2 tablespoons of natural yogurt
- Salt and pepper
- 1 packet of microwavable Mexican rice (250 g packet)
- 2 handfuls of spinach
- 1 small tin of sweetcorn, drained
- 40 g cheddar cheese, grated

Instructions

1. Heat the 1 teaspoon of the oil in a large pan over medium to high heat.
2. Add the chicken on one side and the pepper and onion to the other.
3. Add the fajita seasoning, mix and cook for 5–7 minutes, stirring constantly until cooked through. Remove from the pan when cooked and divide between 2 dishes.
4. When the chicken and veg are cooking, chop the tomatoes, lime and garlic.
5. Get three small bowls, add the avocado to one, tomatoes to one, and yogurt to the last.
6. Season all bowls well with salt and pepper. Squeeze a quarter of lime over the tomatoes and avocado bowls and add the garlic to the yogurt.
7. Heat the rice in the microwave.
8. Arrange the spinach, rice, corn, cheese and lime between the dishes.
9. Add an even amount smashed avocado, tomato salsa and garlic yogurt dip to each dish.

Nutrient Info Per Serving

Calories: 660 | Carbs: 58 g | Fibre: 9 g | Protein: 35 g | Fat: 30 g | Saturated Fat: 8 g

Sun-dried Tomato Pesto Pasta

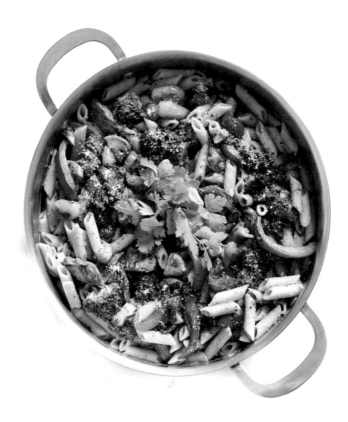

This recipe is a firm favourite with my athletes as it is quick, easy and a tasty fuelling option!

Serves: 2

Time to cook: 20 minutes

Ingredients

- 200 g white penne pasta, uncooked
- 1 teaspoon of extra virgin olive oil
- 2 cloves of garlic, chopped
- 1 medium onion, chopped
- Salt and pepper
- 1 medium chicken breast, diced
- 2 handfuls of mushrooms, chopped
- 2 medium-sized tomatoes, chopped small
- 1 red pepper, chopped
- Handful of broccoli spears, chopped small
- 2 tablespoons of light cream cheese
- 2 teaspoons of sun-dried tomato pesto

Instructions

1. Boil the pasta for 10–13 minutes.
2. Add 1 tablespoon of oil in a pan over low to medium heat.
3. Add the garlic and onion and season with salt and pepper, cook for 5 minutes.
4. Add the chicken and cook for another 5 minutes, then add the mushrooms.
5. Turn up the heat slightly and cook for a further 3 minutes.
6. Add the chopped tomatoes, red pepper and broccoli.
7. Cook for another couple of minutes.
8. Add the cream cheese and the pesto.
9. Stir through the chicken and vegetables for 5 minutes.
10. Drain the pasta (reserve half a cup of pasta water) and add to the pan with the chicken and vegetables.
11. Mix well and add the cup of pasta water.
12. Mix again and divide between 2 dishes.

Nutrient Info Per Serving

Calories: 617 | Carbs: 85 g | Fibre: 11 g | Protein: 37 g | Fat: 12 g | Saturated Fat: 4 g

Quick Egg Fried Rice

This 10-minute, high carbohydrate meal is perfect for when you are in a rush and need to get something cooked quickly. Therefore, I always keep some microwavable rice in the cupboard and frozen veg in the freezer.

Serves: 1

Time to cook: 10 minutes

Vegetarian

Ingredients

- 1 teaspoon of butter
- 2 eggs
- 1 teaspoon of sesame oil
- 2 handfuls of frozen veg
- 1 packet of microwavable long grain rice (250 g packet)
- 1 tablespoon of reduced sodium/light soy sauce
- 1 tablespoon of honey
- Pepper

Instructions

1. Add a large frying pan over medium heat and add the butter.
2. Scramble the eggs and then remove from the pan and set to one side.
3. Add the sesame oil to the pan.
4. Add the frozen veg, season with pepper, and stir fry for 3 minutes.
5. Add the rice and stir fry for 2 minutes.
6. Add the soy sauce and honey, stir fry for 1 min.
7. Add the eggs back into the pan and mix well.
8. Enjoy!

Nutrient Info Per Serving

Calories: 713 | Carbs: 105 g | Fibre: 4 g | Protein: 26 g | Fat: 20 g | Saturated Fat: 4 g

Beetroot and Couscous Wrap

Beetroot is high in nitrates, which have been shown to improve performance. This wrap is the perfect excuse to get them into your training day, and its combination with feta and walnuts makes for a delicious training day meal!

Serves: 1

Time to cook: 5 minutes

Vegan

Ingredients

- 1 large tortilla wrap
- 1 tablespoon of hummus
- Handful of mixed salad leaves
- 100 g cooked couscous
- 4 slices of pickled beetroot, chopped
- 20 g feta cheese, chopped
- 3 walnuts, chopped

Instructions

1. Spread the wrap with hummus.
2. Add your filling along the top half of the wrap, first salad leaves, then couscous, beetroot, feta and chopped walnuts.
3. Fold the sides of the wrap in a little, then holding them firmly, roll the wrap from the top over the filling and towards you.
4. Chop in half and serve.
5. Enjoy!

Nutrient Info Per Serving

Calories: 622 | Carbs: 73 g | Fibre: 8 g | Protein: 22 g | Fat: 25 g | Saturated Fat: 6 g

Taco Fries

Who doesn't love Taco Fries?! The humble spud is a great carb for fuelling and refuelling so I try to create lots of tasty recipes with it. This is a spin on the fast-food option that's much more nutritious but doesn't lack flavour!

Serves: 2

Time to cook: 40 minutes

Ingredients

- 3 medium potatoes (600 g)
- 2 tablespoons of extra virgin olive oil
- Salt and pepper
- 1 onion, diced
- Cloves of garlic, finely diced/crushed
- 1 tablespoon of tomato purée
- 200 g turkey mince
- 2 tablespoon of fajita/taco seasoning
- 1 pepper, chopped
- 1 tin of chopped tomatoes (400 g)
- 40 g cheddar cheese, grated

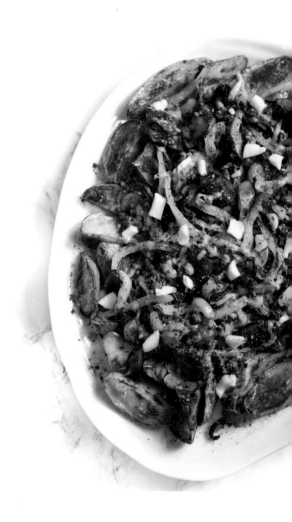

Instructions

1. Preheat oven to 220°C / fan 200°C / 425°F / gas mark 7.
2. Cut the potatoes into fries (about the size of your index finger).
3. Drizzle with a tablespoon of oil, season with salt and pepper and mix well.
4. Cook for 15 minutes, take out and flip the fries to cook evenly, then cook for another 10–15 minutes.
5. While the fries are cooking, heat 1 tablespoon of oil in a pan over a medium heat.
6. Add the onion, garlic, tomato purée and fry for a couple of minutes.
7. Add the turkey mince and mix well, add the fajita/taco seasoning, and mix again. Fry until turkey is cooked through.
8. Add the pepper and tin of tomatoes, bring to the boil, turn down heat and simmer for 7–10 minutes, stirring occasionally.
9. Divide the fries between 2 dishes, add an even amount of the mince mix to each and top with an even amount of cheese.
10. Enjoy!

Nutrient Info Per Serving

Calories: 639 | Carbs: 83 g | Fibre: 13 g | Protein: 41 g | Fat: 11 g | Saturated Fat: 4 g

Easy Veegy Baked Beans

Baked beans are another fuelling food that is massively underrated! They are incredibly versatile and nutritious. I always keep a few tins in the cupboard for a handy fuelling or refuelling option on training days.

Serves: 2

Time to cook: 15 minutes

Vegan

Ingredients

- 100 g white rice, uncooked
- 1 tablespoon of extra virgin olive oil
- 400 g mixed frozen vegetables
- 1 teaspoon of paprika
- 1 tin of baked beans (420 g)
- Salt and pepper

Instructions

1. Cook rice according to packet instructions.
2. Heat the oil over medium heat in a large pan.
3. Add the veg to the pan along with the salt, pepper and paprika, and stir fry for 5–7 minutes.
4. Add the beans, mix well and heat through.
5. Divide the bean mix and rice between 2 dishes.

Nutrient Info Per Serving

Calories: 515 | Carbs: 80 g | Fibre: 16 g | Protein: 21 g | Fat: 9 g | Saturated Fat: 1.3 g

Sweet Potato Toast and Hummus

A quirky spin on beans on toast!

Serves: 6

Time to cook: 20 minutes

Vegan

Ingredients

- 1 medium sweet potato
- Half a tin of mixed beans
- 1 tablespoon of hummus
- 1 handful of spinach
- 1 teaspoon of paprika

Instructions

1. Slice sweet potato into toast-like pieces (about a quarter of an inch thick) and place under the grill.
2. Toast until browned and then flip.
3. Heat the beans up in the bowl in the microwave.
4. Spread each toast slice with hummus.
5. Top with some beans and spinach.
6. Sprinkle the paprika over the top.

Nutrient Info Per Serving

Calories: 572 | Carbs: 77 g | Protein: 17 g | Fat: 18 g | Fibre: 16 g | Saturated Fat: 6 g

Meatball Pasta Bake

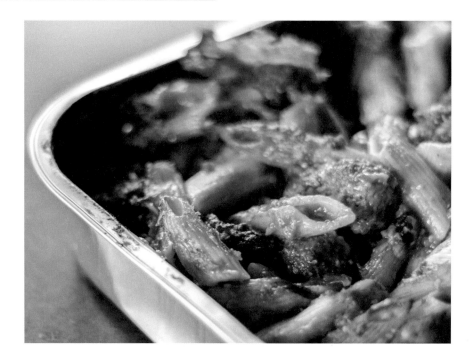

This one takes a bit longer to prepare and cook but it will set you up with a lot of your for the week, and I promise you, it's so tasty it's worth the bit of extra effort!

Serves: 6

Time to cook: 45 minutes

Ingredients

- 300 g extra lean beef mince
- 60 g porridge oats (oatmeal)
- 1 egg
- Salt and pepper
- 3 tablespoons of mixed herbs, dried
- 450 g white pasta (uncooked)
- 1 tablespoon of extra virgin olive oil
- 1 medium onion, chopped
- 4 cloves of garlic, finely chopped/crushed

- 2 medium carrots, peeled and chopped
- 200 g Brussels sprouts, chopped
- 250 g mushrooms, chopped
- Half a head of broccoli, chopped
- 1 pepper, chopped
- 2 tins of chopped tomatoes (400 g each)
- 100 g cheddar cheese, grated

Instructions

1. Make the meatballs by combining the beef mince, porridge, egg, salt, pepper and 1 tablespoon of dried mixed herbs in a bowl. Mix until well combined.
2. Take a small amount of the mix and roll into a meatball (about 2" in diameter), make sure the balls are roughly the same size.
3. When the meatballs are rolled, preheat the oven to 180°C / fan 160°C / 350°F / gas mark 4 and boil the kettle.
4. Put the pasta on to boil (it will only take about 12–15 minutes, don't overcook it).
5. While the pasta is boiling, heat the oil in a very large pan over a medium heat.
6. Add the onion and garlic and cook for 5 minutes, then gently place the meatballs in.
7. While the meatballs are browning, prep the rest of your veg.
8. Add them to the pan as you chop them in the same order: carrot, Brussels sprouts, mushrooms, broccoli, pepper.
9. Gently turn the meatballs as they cook to brown them on all sides.
10. When the meatballs are browned, season the pan well with salt, pepper and 2 tablespoons of mixed herbs.
11. Mix well and then add the 2 tins of tomatoes, mix well again (gently).
12. Add the contents of the pan to a large oven dish.
13. Drain the pasta, add to the pan and mix well.
14. Top with 100 g of grated cheese.
15. Pop the dish into the oven for 10–15 minutes.
16. You should get about 6 portions.

Nutrient Info Per Serving

Calories: 580 | Carbs: 73 g | Fibre: 11 g | Protein: 33 g | Fat: 15 g | Saturated Fat: 6 g

Training Day Dinners

Chicken Fajita Pasta

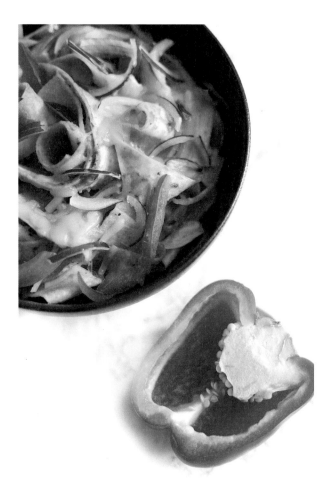

Pasta isn't something you'd often see in Mexican flavoured dishes, but I love mixing things up! As pasta is such an efficient source of fuel, it's important that you keep it interesting, and this dish certainly does that!

Serves: 4

Time to cook: 20 minutes

Ingredients

- 400 g white pasta, uncooked
- 1 tablespoon of extra virgin olive oil
- 5 cloves of garlic, crushed/finely chopped
- 1 onion, chopped
- Salt and pepper
- 200 g chicken breast, chopped
- 60 g Chipotle chilli paste
- 2 bell peppers, chopped
- 2 tablespoons of crème fraîche
- 80 g cheddar cheese, grated

Instructions

1. Boil the pasta for 10–13 minutes.
2. Add 1 tablespoon of oil in a pan over low to medium heat.
3. Add the garlic and onion and season with salt and pepper, cook for 5 minutes.
4. Add the chicken and cook for another 5 minutes, then add the Chipotle chilli paste.
5. Turn up the heat slightly and cook for a further 3 minutes.
6. Add the sliced peppers and cook on low heat until soft, stirring regularly.
7. Add the crème fraîche and stir well, simmer for 5 minutes.
8. Drain the pasta, keep about a quarter of a cup of the pasta water.
9. Add the pasta and reserved pasta water back to the pan.
10. Stir well.
11. Divide between four dishes and top with an even amount of cheese.

Nutrient Info Per Serving

Calories: 611 | Carbs: 77 g | Fibre: 8 g | Protein: 27 g | Fat: 20 g | Saturated Fat: 10 g

Prawn and Coconut Thai Curry

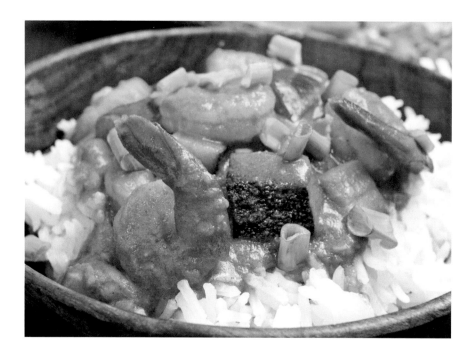

Fuelling meals should never be boring! This recipe is full of flavour and is packed with nutrients.

Serves: 3

Time to cook: 40 minutes

Ingredients

- 200 g basmati rice
- 1 tablespoon of extra virgin olive oil
- 1 medium red onion, chopped
- 4 cloves of garlic, chopped
- 1 thumb sized piece of ginger, grated
- 4 teaspoons of cumin
- 2 teaspoons of coriander (cilantro)
- 1 teaspoon of chilli powder
- 1 teaspoon of turmeric

- Salt and pepper
- 6 medium-sized tomatoes, chopped
- 1 tin of light coconut milk (400 g)
- 200 g spinach
- 400 g peeled and cooked frozen prawns (shrimp)
- 150 g baby corn, halved
- Half a head of broccoli, chopped

Instructions

1. Add 200 g of basmati rice to a bowl and cover with water and soak for 20 minutes. Drain and rinse with cold water, then add to a saucepan and cover with boiling water. Bring to the boil and simmer for 10–12 minutes.
2. Remove lid and leave to stand for 5 minutes.
3. While the rice is cooking, heat the oil in a deep sided frying pan or wok over medium heat.
4. Add the onion, garlic and ginger and cook for 2–3 minutes until softened, but not browned.
5. Add the spices and seasoning and cook for another 1–2 minutes to release the flavours.
6. Add the tomatoes, baby corn, and broccoli. Continue to cook over low heat for another 2 minutes until the tomatoes start to break down. Add the coconut milk and bring to the boil.
7. Mix in the spinach leaves and reduce the heat, continuing to cook until the spinach has collapsed.
8. Add the pawns, sugar and a pinch of salt and cook for a further 2 minutes over a high heat.
9. Lightly fork through the rice and divide the rice and curry evenly between 3 bowls.

Nutrient Info Per Serving

Calories: 608 | Carbs: 70 g | Fibre: 10 g | Protein: 35 g | Fat: 17 g | Saturated Fat: 9 g

Basil Pesto Spaghetti

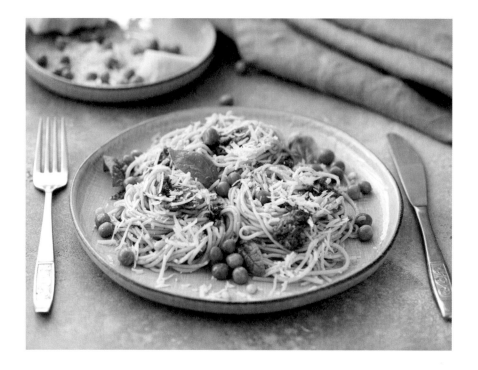

This a simple, speedy recipe perfect for when you're in a rush but want to ensure you're fuelling or refuelling optimally!

Serves: 2

Time to cook: 15 minutes

Ingredients

- 200 g white spaghetti (uncooked)
- 1 teaspoon of extra virgin olive oil
- 150 g turkey steak, diced
- 1 medium pepper, chopped
- Salt and pepper
- 200 g frozen peas
- 1 tablespoon of basil pesto
- 1 teaspoon of pine nuts

Instructions

1. Boil the spaghetti for 10–13 minutes.
2. When the spaghetti is cooking, add the oil in a pan over medium heat.
3. Add the turkey and cook for a couple of minutes.
4. Add the pepper and season with salt and pepper, cook for 3–5 minutes.
5. Add the peas.
6. Cook for another couple of minutes.
7. Add the pesto.
8. Stir through the turkey and vegetables.
9. Drain the spaghetti and add it back to the pan.
10. Mix well and divide between 2 dishes.
11. Toast the pine nuts in a small saucepan until lightly browned (keep a close eye when toasting as they burn easily).
12. Top each dish with an even amount of the nuts.

Nutrient Info Per Serving

Calories: 632 | Carbs: 82 g | Fibre: 11 g | Protein: 39 g | Fat: 14 g | Saturated Fat: 3 g

Prawn Massaman Curry

Making a curry paste from scratch doesn't have to be a daunting task. Using a smoothie blitzer will make for an easy clean up and, with the right ingredients, you'll have a delicious curry paste in seconds!

Serves: 4

Time to cook: 40 minutes

Ingredients

- 250 g basmati rice
- 1 teaspoon of butter
- 400 g prawns, cooked and frozen (shrimp)
- 1 tin of light coconut milk
- 1 heaped teaspoon of flour
- 1 vegetable stock cube
- 1 cup of water
- 400 g baby potatoes, quartered
- 1 lemon, juiced
- 20 g fresh coriander (cilantro)
- 1 courgette (zucchini), chopped
- 250 g green beans
- 1 medium pepper, chopped

For the Massaman sauce
- 1 onion, chopped
- 4 garlic cloves
- 2 tbsp Massaman curry paste
- 2 red chillies, deseeded and roughly chopped
- 1 tsp ground cinnamon
- 1 tbsp ground cumin
- 1 tsp dried coriander (cilantro)
- 2 tsp salt
- 1 tsp black pepper

Instructions

1. Cook the basmati rice according to packet instructions.
2. Add all the ingredients for the Massaman sauce to a blender or food processor and blitz into a paste.
3. Put a large saucepan over a medium heat and melt the butter. Add the prawns and cook for 2 minutes, stirring occasionally with a spatula. Remove and set to one side.
4. Reduce the heat and add the Massaman sauce. Cook gently for 2–3 minutes.
5. Add the coconut milk, flour, vegetable stock cube, salt and water and stir thoroughly, then cover and simmer for 5 minutes.
6. Remove the lid and add the potatoes, mixing in thoroughly. Place the lid back on and simmer for a further 15–20 minutes until the potatoes are soft.
7. Once the potatoes have been cooking for 10 minutes, add the courgette, pepper, and green beans.
8. Add the lemon juice and coriander to the curry, give it one final mix, then serve alongside the basmati rice.

Nutrient Info Per Serving

Calories: 585 | **Carbs: 82 g** | **Fibre: 11 g** | **Protein: 30 g** | **Fat: 13 g** | **Saturated Fat: 8 g**

Chilli Con Carne

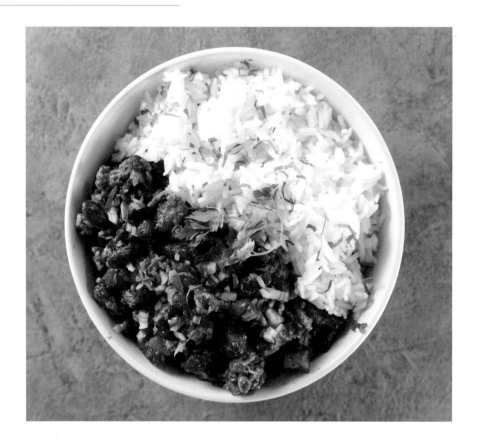

Who doesn't love this classic recipe? The combination of rice and beans make for an excellent fuelling combination, and this recipe is high in iron and vitamin C!

Serves: 2

Time to cook: 30 minutes

Ingredients

- 120 g long grain rice, uncooked
- 1 tablespoon of extra virgin olive oil
- 1 small onion, chopped
- 2 cloves of garlic, finely diced/crushed
- 1 teaspoon chilli powder
- 1 teaspoon paprika
- 1 teaspoon cumin
- Salt and pepper
- 150 g lean 5% minced beef
- 1 tablespoon of tomato purée
- Half a beef stock cube
- Half a tin of chopped tomatoes (200 g)
- 1 teaspoon sugar
- 1 pepper, chopped
- 1 tin of kidney beans, drained

Instructions

1. Boil the kettle and cook the rice according to packet instructions.
2. While the rice is cooking, heat the oil over a medium heat in a large saucepan.
3. Add the onion, garlic, all the seasoning and cook gently for 5 minutes.
4. Add the beef and tomato purée, crumble in half the beef stock cube and cook until the beef is browned. Drain off any excess liquid.
5. Add the tinned tomatoes and sugar, bring to the boil, then reduce the heat and simmer for 10 minutes, then add the chopped pepper and the beans for the last 5 minutes. Stir regularly.
6. When the rice is cooked, divide between two dishes and top with half the chilli on each.

Nutrient Info Per Serving

Calories: 561 | Carbs: 82 g | Fibre: 17 g | Protein: 33 g | Fat: 6 g | Saturated Fat: 2 g

Tomato Pasta Bake

Batch cooking some meals and freezing them will ensure you always have a good fuelling meal at the ready, even on days when you are tight for time or dealing with a busy schedule!

Serves: 5

Time to cook: 45 minutes

Ingredients

- 1 tablespoon of extra virgin olive oil
- 1 onion, diced
- 2 cloves of garlic, finely diced
- 300 g chicken breast, diced
- 1 tin of chopped tomatoes, 400 g
- 1 teaspoon of sugar
- 1 tablespoon of Worcestershire sauce
- Salt and pepper
- 500 g white pasta, uncooked
- Half a head of broccoli, chopped
- 1 courgette (zucchini), chopped
- 60 g cheddar cheese, grated
- 1 tablespoon of dried mixed herbs

Instructions

1. Preheat the oven to 180°C / fan 160°C / 350°F / gas mark 4.
2. Heat the oil in a medium pan and fry the onion for 5 minutes until soft.
3. Add the garlic and mixed herbs, cook for a further minute.
4. Add the chicken and cook for 3–5 minutes.
5. Mix in the tomatoes and sugar, bring to the boil and simmer for 10 minutes.

6. Add a few dashes of Worcestershire sauce and season with salt and pepper.
7. Meanwhile, cook the pasta according to pack instructions.
8. Drain the pasta and stir into the sauce.
9. Add the broccoli and courgette and mix well.
10. Add to a large baking dish.
11. Scatter over the cheese and bake for 10 minutes.

Nutrient Info Per Serving

Calories: 669 | Carbs: 104 g | Protein: 31 g | Fat: 11 g | Fibre: 13 g | Saturated Fat: 4 g

Jerk Chicken with Beans and Rice

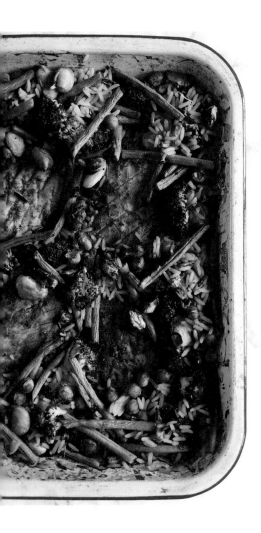

A good spice cabinet is the key to flavoursome meals! Jerk seasoning tastes amazing with chicken, and this dish is worth the marinating time!

Serves: 4

Time to cook: 30 minutes (not including marinating time)

Ingredients

- 2 tablespoons of extra virgin olive oil
- 4 teaspoons of Jerk seasoning
- Salt and pepper
- 4 boneless chicken thighs
- 1 medium onion, diced
- 250 g long grain rice, uncooked
- Half a chicken stock cube
  (make 500 mL stock)
- 250 g green beans, topped and tailed
- 1 tin of mixed beans, drained
- 100 g broccoli, chopped
- 200 g frozen peas

Instructions

1. In a large bowl, whisk together the olive oil, 3 teaspoons of Jerk seasoning, a pinch of salt and a pinch of pepper. Add the chicken and toss to coat well. Cover with plastic wrap and marinate in the refrigerator for at least 30 minutes, up to 4 hours.
2. Remove the chicken from the marinade and place in a large pot/pan (with a lid) over a medium-high heat, being careful not to overcrowd the pot/pan.
3. Cook for 3 minutes or until golden brown, then flip and repeat on the other side. Remove the chicken from the pot and set aside (it doesn't have to be cooked through at this stage, only browned on each side).
4. Add the onion to the pot/pan. Cook for 2–3 minutes, or until starting to soften.
5. Add the rice and chicken stock. Season with the remaining teaspoon of Jerk seasoning. Bring to a boil, then return the chicken thighs to the pot.
6. Cover with a lid and simmer for 12–15 minutes (or until the rice is cooked).
7. For the last 7 minutes of cooking, add the green beans, tin of drained beans, broccoli and peas and stir through (try not to move the chicken around too much).
8. Divide between 4 dishes.

Nutrient Info Per Serving

Calories: 578 | Carbs: 67 g | Fibre: 11 g | Protein: 34 g | Fat: 17 g | Saturated Fat: 4 g

Spiced Carrot and Lentil Soup

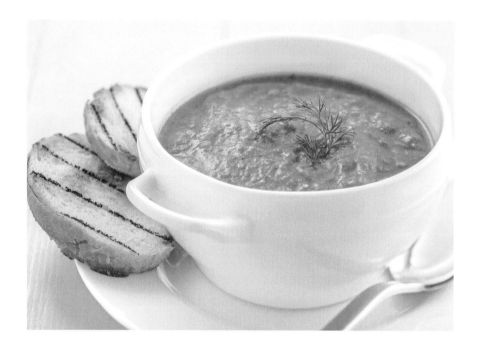

I always insist that healthy cooking doesn't have to be expensive, and this recipe is a testament to that! A tasty soup is always my go-to option for fuelling on those cold winter nights and, with a little added spice, this recipe will heat you up even more.

Serves: 5

Time to cook: 40 minutes

Vegan

Ingredients

- 1 teaspoon of extra virgin olive oil
- 1 medium onion, chopped
- 6 cloves of garlic
- 1 tablespoon of paprika
- 2 teaspoons of turmeric
- 1 teaspoon of cumin
- 1 teaspoon of cinnamon
- 1 teaspoon of coriander powder (cilantro)
- Salt and pepper
- 10 medium carrots, peeled and chopped
- 2 tins of chopped tomatoes
- 300 g red split lentils
- 1 vegetable stock cube (make 1 L stock)

Instructions

1. Heat the oil over a high heat in a very large saucepan (the biggest you can get your hands on!).
2. Add the onion and garlic, fry for a couple of minutes.
3. Add all the spices, salt and pepper, and cook for 30 seconds.
4. Add the carrots and cook for 2 minutes.
5. Add the tomatoes, lentils and stock.
6. Bring to the boil, then reduce the heat and simmer for 15 minutes.
7. When the soup is done, set aside to cool for 10 minutes. If you want a smooth soup, use a stick (handheld) blender or blender to blitz the soup – if you don't have either of those don't worry, you can just have a chunky soup!
8. Divide between 5 dishes.

Nutrient Info Per Serving

Calories: 352 | Carbs: 53 g | Fibre: 12 g | Protein: 19 g | Fat: 4 g | Saturated Fat: 0.4 g

Nutrient Info Per Serving (with two slices of white bread)

Calories: 564 | Carbs: 92 g | Fibre: 14 g | Protein: 28 g | Fat: 6 g | Saturated Fat: 4 g

Taco Mince and Rice

By using precooked rice and ready-made seasoning we can cut down on the amount of time we have to cook and still get a nutritious, tasty meal!

Serves: 2

Time to cook: 20 minutes

Ingredients

- 1 tablespoon of extra virgin olive oil
- 1 small onion, chopped
- 3 cloves of garlic, finely diced/crushed
- 2 tablespoons of taco seasoning
- 100 g turkey mince
- 2 handfuls of mushrooms, chopped
- 3 medium tomatoes
- 1 pepper, chopped
- 1 small tin of sweetcorn, drained
- 1 tin of kidney beans, drained
- 1 packet of microwavable long grain rice (250 g each)
- 40 g cheddar cheese, grated
- Salt and pepper

Instructions

1. Heat the oil in a deep sided frying pan over a medium heat.
2. Add the onions and garlic and cook for 2–3 minutes until softened, but not browned. Add the taco seasoning and cook for another 1–2 minutes to release the flavours.
3. Add the mince and mushrooms, cook for 2–3 minutes.

4. Add the tomatoes and continue to cook over a low heat for another 2 minutes until the tomatoes start to break down. Add the pepper.
5. Add the sweetcorn and beans and mix well.
6. Add the packet of rice and mix.
7. Divide the mince and rice mix evenly between 2 bowls. Top with an even amount of cheese.

Nutrient Info Per Serving

Calories: 641 | **Carbs: 77 g** | **Fibre: 16 g** | **Protein: 34 g** | **Fat: 18 g** | **Saturated Fat: 6 g**

Ham and Pea Risotto

Risotto can be a bit of a daunting recipe as it requires a little time and attention to cook. However, I've cheated a little, and we're going to do it the speedy way in this recipe!

Serves: 2

Time to cook: 20 minutes

Ingredients

- 1 small onion, finely diced
- 1 garlic clove, finely diced/crushed
- 160 g Arborio risotto rice, uncooked
- 1 tablespoon of Bouillon Paste, make 300 mL stock
- 2 teaspoons extra virgin olive oil
- 200 g frozen peas
- 80 g cooked ham, crumbled/chopped
- 2 tablespoons of fresh parmesan, grated
- Salt and pepper

Instructions

1. Peel and dice the onion and peel the garlic.
2. Cook rice in vegetable stock for 15–20 minutes. Keep stirring regularly.
3. Meanwhile, heat the oil in a wide pan, cook the onions and garlic for 5–7 minutes, then add frozen peas and slices of ham. Cook for a further 2 minutes.
4. Take the peas and ham off the heat and transfer to the rice with some cheese (leave some behind for garnish) and mix well to combine all the ingredients.
5. Remove from heat and serve in a bowl. Sprinkle remaining cheese, season with salt and pepper to taste.

Nutrient Info Per Serving

Calories: 555 | Carbs: 77 g | Fibre: 7 g | Protein: 28 g | Fat: 14 g | Saturated Fat: 5 g

Chapter 9

Recovery Day Recipes

Recovery Day Breakfasts

Breakfast Burrito

One of my favourite recovery day recipes. High in healthy fats, protein and fibre, this breakfast is packed with nutrients to help you recover!

Servings: 1

Time to make: 10 minutes

Ingredients

- 15 g (2") of chorizo, chopped
- 1 egg
- Salt and pepper
- 1 whole wheat wrap
- 2 tablespoons of baked beans, heated
- Half an avocado, mashed
- 1 spring onions/scallion, chopped
- 1 handful of spinach
- 1 tablespoon of hot sauce
- Half of a teaspoon of fajita seasoning

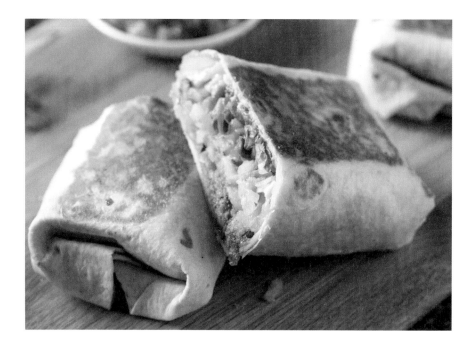

Instructions

1. Heat a large non-stick pan over a medium-high heat.
2. Add the chorizo and cook, breaking it up until it is slightly crisp for about 5 minutes. Remove to a paper towel-lined plate using a slotted spoon. Wipe the pan clean and return to the heat.
3. Beat the egg in a medium bowl until frothy. Sprinkle with salt and pepper.
4. Add the eggs to the pan, keep stirring until the eggs are fluffy and just set. This should take about 3 minutes. Remove from the pan and keep warm. Wipe out the pan and return it to the heat.
5. Warm the wrap in the pan
6. Heat the beans in the microwave for 1 minute.
7. Build the burrito by layering the avocado, scrambled egg, beans, chorizo, scallions, spinach and hot sauce. Sprinkle over the fajita seasoning.
8. Fold in the two sides and roll up tightly.
9. Cut in half, enjoy!

Nutrient Info Per Serving

Calories: 580 | Carbs: 43 g | Fibre: 11 g | Protein: 25 g | Fat: 32 g | Saturated Fat: 8 g

Omelette

Simple, tasty and effective. If you mess it up, just give it a good mix and pretend you were making scrambled eggs!

Servings: 1

Time to make: 10 minutes

Vegetarian

Ingredients

- 3 eggs
- 1 teaspoon of extra virgin olive oil
- Handful of mushrooms, chopped
- Handful of cherry tomatoes, chopped
- 30 g cheddar cheese, grated
- Salt and pepper

Instructions

1. Whisk the eggs in a bowl until they're combined and there are no large blobs of white still separate (or you'll end up with a blotchy omelette). Season with salt and pepper.
2. Heat the oil in a frying pan.
3. Fry off the chopped veg for a few minutes.
4. Add the eggs in one go and swirl and shake the pan so they cover the surface.
5. As soon as the eggs start to set, pull the edges of the omelette into the centre of the pan and shake the pan so any liquid egg spills into the gaps. Add the cheese. Your omelette is ready when the centre is still slightly liquid – it will continue to cook when you fold it over.
6. Fold the omelette in half as you slide it onto a plate or fold the two sides in and then tip it in half as it goes onto the plate to make a neat oblong shape.

Nutrient Info Per Serving

Calories: 446 | Carbs: 9 g | Fibre: 2 g | Protein: 32 g | Fat: 30 g | Saturated Fat: 12 g

Lighter Fry Up

Growing up in Ireland, Sunday mornings usually consisted of a fry up with my family. However, with overconsumption of processed meats linked with negative health issues, I've redesigned the classic fry up to be more nutrient-dense.

Servings: 1

Time to make: 20 minutes

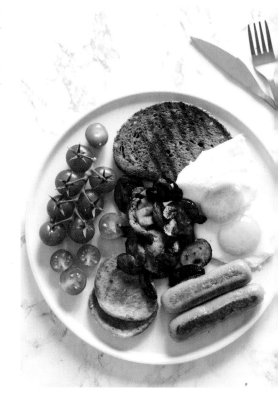

Ingredients

- 2 turkey sausages
- 2 bacon medallions
- Handful of mushrooms, chopped
- 1 teaspoon of extra virgin olive oil
- 2 eggs
- Handful of cherry tomatoes, chopped
- 1 slice of wholegrain toast, lightly buttered
- Salt and pepper

Instructions

1. Grill the sausages and bacon under a medium heat. The bacon will take about 3–4 minutes on each side; the sausages will take about 5–6 minutes on each side.
2. While the meat is cooking, fry the mushrooms in the olive oil over a medium heat, season with salt and pepper.
3. Cook the eggs however you like (don't forget to season with salt and pepper) and toast your bread.
4. Grab a large plate and add your toast, eggs, chopped cherry tomatoes, sausages, bacon, and mushrooms.
5. Enjoy!

Nutrient Info Per Serving

Calories: 592 | **Carbs:** 25 g | **Fibre:** 5 g | **Protein:** 49 g | **Fat:** 32 g | **Saturated Fat:** 10 g

Chickpea and Avo Toast

This recipe is a great option if you want a break from eggs but still want to keep protein high for breakfast. It is a simple, but nutrient-dense recipe and even looks a little fancy!

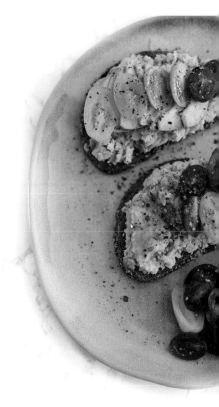

Servings: 1

Time to make: 10 minutes

Vegan

Ingredients

- 2 slices of wholegrain bread, toasted
- Half a tin of chickpeas (400 g), drained
- Salt and pepper
- Half an avocado, mashed
- Handful of cherry tomatoes, halved
- Sprinkle of chilli flakes
- 1 teaspoon of extra virgin olive oil

Instructions

1. While the bread is toasting, heat the chickpeas in a bowl in the microwave for 1 minute.
2. Mash and season with salt and pepper.
3. In a second bowl, mash the avocado and season with salt and pepper.
4. Spread the chickpeas on each slice of toast and top with an even amount of avocado.
5. Top each slice with halved cherry tomatoes.
6. Sprinkle with chilli flakes and drizzle with olive oil.

Nutrient Info Per Serving

Calories: 508 | Carbs: 49 g | Fibre: 14 g | Protein: 20 g | Fat: 23 g | Saturated Fat: 4 g

Egg Cups

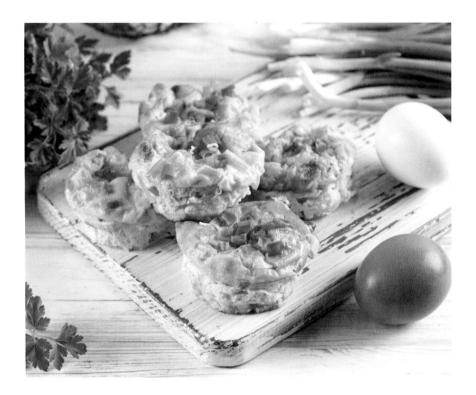

These are a great grab and go option for your recovery day mornings. Keep them in the fridge and reheat in the microwave for a delicious, nutritious breakfast. They also work great as a high protein snack!

Servings: 4 (3 egg cups = 1 serving)

Time to make: 30 minutes

Vegetarian

Ingredients

* 10 eggs
* 50 mL milk
* Salt and pepper
* 1 teaspoon of extra virgin olive oil

Toppings
* Half a pepper, chopped
* 20 g cheddar cheese, grated
* Handful of mushrooms, chopped
* Handful of cherry tomatoes, chopped
* 150 g broccoli, chopped small
* Handful of spinach leaves, chopped

Instructions

1. Preheat oven to 180°C / fan 160°C / 350°F / gas mark 4.
2. Add eggs, milk, salt and pepper to a bowl and whisk.
3. Rub a 12-hole muffin tin with the olive oil.
4. Pour an equal amount of the egg mix into each hole.
5. Divide the toppings as you wish between each hole.
6. Bake for 15 minutes.
7. Keep in the fridge in an airtight container for 5 days.

Nutrient Info Per Serving

Calories: 252 | Carbs: 6 g | Fibre: 3 g | Protein: 22 g | Fat: 15 g | Saturated Fat: 4 g

Hot Rosti

Potatoes for breakfast, what's not to love! Rostis are delicious, and the combination of hot sauce, sour cream, egg and avocado takes this dish to the next level!

Servings: 2

Time to make: 30 minutes

Vegetarian

Ingredients

- 2 small potatoes
- 2 tablespoons of plain flour
- Salt and pepper
- Half a small red onion, diced
- Half a teaspoon of paprika
- 2 scallions, finely chopped
- Fresh coriander (cilantro), 10 sprigs, chopped
- 3 eggs
- 1 avocado, sliced
- 2 tablespoons of reduced fat sour cream
- 1 lime, juiced
- 2 teaspoons of hot sauce
- 1 tablespoon of extra virgin olive oil

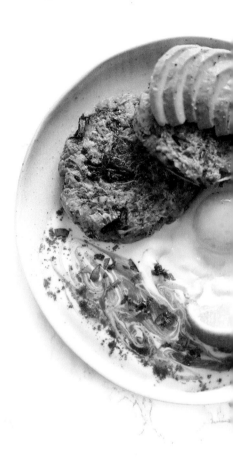

Instructions

1. Peel and grate the potatoes, wrap in a clean tea towel and squeeze out as much liquid as you can. Add the grated potato to a bowl.
2. Stir in the flour, salt, red onion, paprika, scallions, coriander (save a little of this for garnish) and 1 egg. Mix well.
3. Heat the oil in a pan. Add half the rosti mix, flatten it down evenly with a spatula.
4. Fry for 3–4 minutes (until golden brown), then flip over and fry on the other side for another 3 minutes until golden brown.
5. Remove the rosti from the pan with a spatula and set on some paper towels to drain off any oil.
6. Repeat with the other half of the mix.
7. When the second rosti is cooked, add the remaining eggs and fry to your liking.
8. Add each rosti to a plate, top with the fried eggs, half an avocado, a tablespoon of sour cream, a drizzle of lime juice and hot sauce and a few sprigs of coriander.

Nutrient Info Per Serving

Calories: 577 | **Carbs: 49 g** | **Fibre: 7 g** | **Protein: 20 g** | **Fat: 32 g** | **Saturated Fat: 9 g**

Rushing Around Breakfast Baked Bars

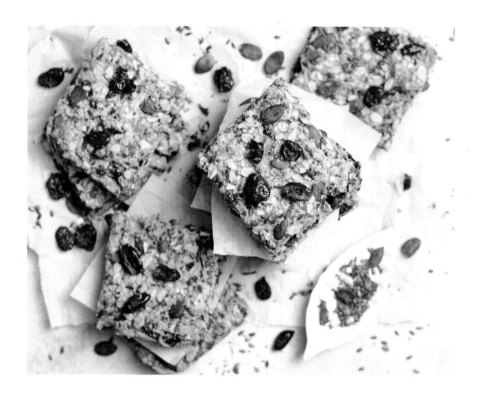

Perfect for those who need to roll out of bed and out the door but still want to get some nutrients in on the go! Packed full of healthy fats and slow-releasing carbs, these bars can be used as a snack option as well.

Servings: 12 bars

Time to make: 30 minutes

Vegetarian

Ingredients

- 100 g peanut butter
- 100 g honey
- 150 g oats
- 150 g mixed nuts
- 100 g blueberries, dried
- 100 g cranberries, dried
- 4 tablespoons of chia seeds
- 4 tablespoons of sunflower seeds
- 1 teaspoon of cinnamon

Instructions

1. Preheat the oven to 150°C / fan 130°C / 300°F / gas mark.
2. Heat the peanut butter and honey in a small pan and stir until melted.
3. Add the dry ingredients to a bowl and mix.
4. Add the honey/peanut butter mix to the dry ingredients and mix well.
5. Press the mix into a non-stick (or line it with greaseproof paper) oven dish (to whatever thickness you like).
6. Pop it into the oven for at least 15–20 minutes (keep an eye that it doesn't burn).
7. Let cool completely and cut into 12 bars, roughly the same size.
8. Store in the fridge for up to a week, or the freezer for up to a month.

Nutrient Info Per Serving (per bar)

Calories: 278 | Carbs: 23 g | Fibre: 5 g | Protein: 7 g | Fat: 16 g | Saturated Fat: 2 g

Veggie Breakfast

This brunch option is packed full of different foods and flavour! With nearly 5 portions of veg and over 30 g protein, this is a perfect recovery meal for players.

Servings: 1

Time to make: 25 minutes

Vegetarian

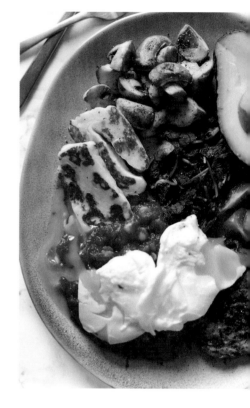

Ingredients

- 1 hash brown
- 40 g of halloumi, sliced
- 2 eggs
- 1 teaspoon of butter
- 1 handful of mushrooms, sliced
- 1 handful of spinach
- 1 medium tomato
- 2 tablespoons of baked beans
- Quarter of an avocado

Instructions

1. Cook the hash brown in the oven (according to packet instructions) and grill the halloumi until browned on both sides.
2. To poach the egg, please see chapter 6.
3. Heat the butter in a small pan and cook the mushrooms and spinach. As they are cooking, cut the tomato in half and fry on each side until browned.
4. Heat the beans in the microwave.
5. When all ingredients are cooked, add them all to a large plate with the avocado, and enjoy!

Nutrient Info Per Serving

Calories: 623 | Carbs: 33 g | Fibre: 9 g | Protein: 33 g | Fat: 38 g | Saturated Fat: 16 g

Smoothie Bowl

A 5-minute breakfast that is absolutely packed with vitamins, minerals, high in fibre and protein – did I mention it's delicious? You can get inventive with smoothie bowls and mix and match the toppings!

Servings: 1

Time to make: 5 minutes

Vegetarian

Ingredients

- 3 tablespoons of low-fat Greek yogurt
- 2 handfuls of frozen blueberries
- 1 tablespoon of almond butter
- 1 banana
- 20 g cashew nuts
- 1 teaspoon flax seeds
- 1 teaspoon pumpkin seeds
- 1 apple, sliced
- Handful of raspberries
- 1 teaspoon of honey

Instructions

1. Blitz the yogurt, blueberries, almond butter and banana, then add to a large bowl.
2. Top with the cashew nuts, seeds, sliced apple and berries.
3. Drizzle the honey over the top.

Nutrient Info Per Serving

Calories: 569 | **Carbs:** 60 g | **Fibre:** 11 g | **Protein:** 26 g | **Fat:** 22 g | **Saturated Fat:** 3 g

Egg Galette

This is something different to the usual recovery breakfast, but is easier to make than it looks! Use a roll of puff pastry for this recipe and try to cut it to the size I've recommended.

Servings: 2

Time to make: 25 minutes

Vegetarian

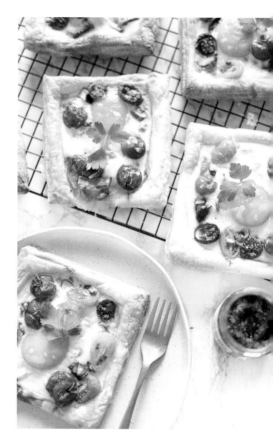

Ingredients

- 2 squares of puff pastry (about 50 g)
- 1 pepper, chopped
- Handful of cherry tomatoes
- Handful of mushrooms
- 2 tablespoons of sun-dried tomato pesto
- 2 eggs
- Salt and pepper
- 60 g feta cheese, chopped into small cubes

Instructions

1. If time permits, defrost the pastry in the refrigerator and ensure the pastry remains chilled.
2. Preheat your oven to 220°C / fan 200°C / 425°F / gas mark 7.
3. Line two trays with baking paper. Cut your pastry into squares that are approximately 12.5 cm/5" on each side. It is easier to assemble pastries on the baking tray.
4. Chop the veg to your liking.
5. Fold in the edges of each square of pastry about 1 inch on every edge.

6. Spread a tablespoon of sun-dried tomato pesto over each square.
7. Distribute the feta, tomatoes, pepper, and mushrooms evenly on the puff pastry squares, leaving a space in the middle of each square.
8. Crack an egg into the space in the middle, season with salt and pepper.
9. Brush the edges of the pastry with beaten egg.
10. Bake for 15 minutes, or until golden on the top and bottom of the pastry.

Nutrient Info Per Serving

Calories: 471 | Carbs: 25 g | Fibre: 5 g | Protein: 18 g | Fat: 32 g | Saturated Fat: 13 g

Recovery Day Lunches

Recovery Bowl

On recovery days we know our big focus is on consuming varied, nutrient-dense foods – this dish is the epitome of this aim! It boasts 6 portions of veg, high protein, high fibre and healthy fats. Make it a once-a-week meal!

Servings: 1

Time to make: 30 minutes

Ingredients

- 4 teaspoons of extra virgin olive oil
- Half a medium sweet potato, diced
- Salt and pepper
- 1 teaspoon of paprika
- 100 g turkey steak, diced
- 2 handfuls of chopped broccoli
- Handful of mushrooms, chopped
- Handful of spinach
- Handful of cherry tomatoes, chopped
- Half an avocado, chopped

Instructions

1. Preheat the oven to 220°C / fan 200°C / 425°F / gas mark 7.
2. Drizzle 1 teaspoon of oil over the sweet potato and season with salt, pepper and half a teaspoon of paprika. Mix well.
3. Bake for about 15 minutes but check regularly.
4. Heat 1 teaspoon of oil in a pan over medium heat.
5. Season the turkey with salt, pepper and half a teaspoon of paprika, add to the pan and cook for about 3–4 minutes on each side. Ensure it is cooked through.

6. Add the broccoli and mushrooms to another baking tray, drizzle with 1 teaspoon of oil. Season with salt and pepper. Mix well.
7. Put in the oven and cook for about 10 minutes, check regularly and mix.
8. Add the spinach, tomatoes and avocado to a bowl.
9. Add the turkey to the bowl.
10. Add the sweet potato and vegetables once cooked.

Nutrient Info Per Serving

Calories: 571 | Carbs: 31 g | Fibre: 10 g | Protein: 33 g | Fat: 33 g | Saturated Fat: 6 g

Chicken Fajita Salad

This dish focuses on protein, healthy fats and vegetables. However, if you want to increase the carbs, you can add the chicken, veg and avocado to some tortilla wraps!

Servings: 2

Time to make: 20 minutes (not including marinating time)

Ingredients

- 2 teaspoons of extra virgin olive oil
- 1 lime, juiced
- 1 teaspoon of coriander (cilantro)
- 1 garlic clove, finely diced/crushed
- 1 teaspoon of sugar
- 1 teaspoon of chilli flakes
- 1 teaspoon of cumin
- Salt and pepper
- 400 g chicken breast, sliced
- 1 small red onion, sliced
- 1 pepper, sliced
- 2 large handfuls of chopped lettuce
- 1 avocado, mashed

Instructions

1. To make the dressing/marinade, whisk olive oil, lime juice, coriander, garlic, sugar, chilli flakes, cumin, salt and pepper in a bowl.
2. Place the chicken in a separate bowl and pour over half the dressing/marinade. Coat the chicken well, cover the bowl and place in the fridge for 30 minutes.
3. When the chicken is ready, heat a large pan over a medium-high heat and add the chicken, cook, then remove from the pan and set to one side.
4. Add the red onion and sliced pepper to the pan, cook on high for 5 minutes, stirring all the time until soft.

5. Add the lettuce to 2 plates.
6. Top each salad with half the chicken and veggies.
7. Serve with reserved dressing and top with an even amount of mashed avocado.

Nutrient Info Per Serving

Calories: 466 | Carbs: 14 g | Fibre: 7 g | Protein: 51 g | Fat: 21 g | Saturated Fat: 4 g

Peri Peri Chicken Pitta

You can choose how hot you want your
peri peri sauce for this recipe!

Servings: 1

Time to make: 20 minutes

Ingredients

- Half a medium chicken breast,
  sliced
- 1 tablespoon of peri peri sauce
- 50 g halloumi cheese, sliced
- 1 wholemeal pitta bread
- 2 teaspoons of red onion
  chutney/relish
- 1 tablespoon of garlic mayonnaise
- 1 tomato, sliced
- 1 large handful of chopped
  lettuce

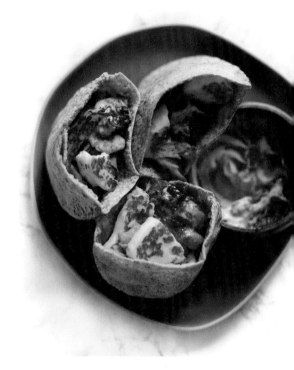

Instructions

1. Slice the chicken into strips and toss in the peri peri sauce. Heat the grill to
   high, grill on all sides for 10–12 minutes in total or until cooked through and
   a little charred.
2. Fry off the halloumi slices until browned on each side.
3. Warm the pitta in a toaster.
4. Slice the pittas in half, spread with the relish and garlic mayo, add the chicken
   and top with the halloumi, tomato and lettuce.

Nutrient Info Per Serving

Calories: 499 | Carbs: 43 g | Fibre: 5 g | Protein: 37 g | Fat: 18 g | Saturated Fat: 9 g

Prawn and Mango Salad

This is a summer lunch favourite of mine. It's quick, full of flavour and uses a combination of ingredients that work incredibly well together! If you have never cut a mango, please do a quick google, you'll thank me later!

Servings: 2

Time to make: 15 minutes

Ingredients

- 1 tablespoon of extra virgin olive oil
- 1 lime, juiced
- Salt and pepper
- 20 g pine nuts, toasted
- 200 g prawns, peeled and cooked (shrimp)
- 1 mango, chopped
- 1 pepper, chopped
- 2 handfuls of cherry tomatoes, quartered
- 2 handfuls of spinach, chopped
- Half an avocado, chopped
- Half a ball of buffalo mozzarella, chopped

Instructions

1. Add the oil and lime juice to a bowl. Season well with salt and pepper and whisk well.
2. Toast the pine nuts on a pan over medium heat and toast. They will burn easily, so be careful.
3. Add all other ingredients to a large bowl and mix well.
4. Add the dressing and mix well.
5. Divide between 2 dishes and top with an equal amount of pine nuts.

Nutrient Info Per Serving

Calories: 464 | Carbs: 22 g | Fibre: 5 g | Protein: 37 g | Fat: 27 g | Saturated Fat: 8 g

Mexican Quinoa

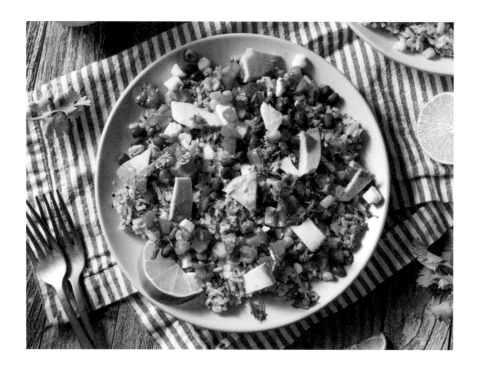

I urge you to make this meal if you've never had a vegan dish before!

Servings: 2

Time to make: 15 minutes

Vegan

Ingredients

- Half a vegetable stock cube (makes 300 mL of stock)
- 100 g quinoa, uncooked
- 1 teaspoon of extra virgin olive oil
- 1 clove of garlic, finely chopped/diced
- 1 teaspoon of chilli powder
- 1 teaspoon of cumin
- 1 tin of red kidney beans, drained
- 1 small tin of sweetcorn, drained
- 2 handfuls of cherry tomatoes, halved
- 1 avocado, chopped
- Half a lime, cut in half again
- Pepper

Instructions

1. Bring the stock to a boil in a medium saucepan and add the quinoa, simmer for 10 minutes.
2. While the quinoa is cooking, heat the oil in a medium saucepan over medium heat.
3. Add the garlic, pepper, and spices and cook for a couple of minutes.
4. Add the kidney beans and sweetcorn, mix well.
5. Cook for 5 minutes and then turn the heat right down.
6. When the quinoa is cooked, drain as much of the liquid as possible from it.
7. Add to the beans, sweetcorn and tomatoes at this point and mix well.
8. Divide between 2 dishes with an equal amount of the avocado on both with a wedge of lime.

Nutrient Info Per Serving

Calories: 458 | Carbs: 56 g | Fibre: 18 g | Protein: 18 g | Fat: 14 g | Saturated Fat: 2 g

Bridge Nutrition Pasta Bake

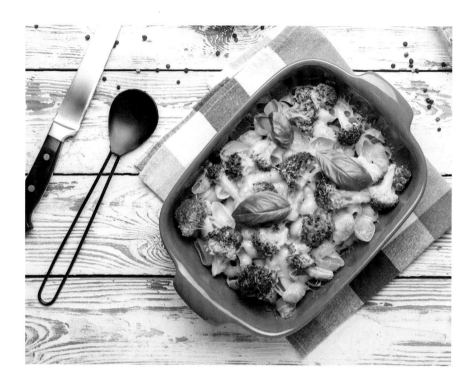

A great dish if you must still be active on your days off to ensure you are prepped to recover well between intense sessions.

Servings: 4

Time to make: 15 minutes

Ingredients

- 250 g whole wheat pasta (uncooked)
- 2 tablespoons of extra virgin olive oil
- 5 cloves of garlic, chopped
- 1 onion, chopped
- 300 g chicken, diced
- 250 g mushrooms, chopped
- Salt and pepper
- 1 head of broccoli, chopped small
- 250 g single fresh cream
- 50 g breadcrumbs
- 60 g reduced fat cheese

Instructions

1. Preheat the oven to 220°C / fan 200°C / 425°F / gas mark 7.
2. Cook the pasta according to packet instructions.
3. While the pasta is cooking, heat oil in a large pan over medium heat and fry the garlic and onion for 2 minutes or until soft.
4. Add the chicken and mushrooms and cook for 5 minutes.
5. Season well with salt and pepper.
6. Add the broccoli and cook for 2 minutes, keep stirring regularly.
7. Add the cream and simmer for a couple of minutes.
8. Add the pasta to a large oven dish, add the mix from the pan on top and stir well.
9. Top with breadcrumbs and cheese.
10. Pop into the oven and bake for 10 minutes.
11. Divide between 4 dishes.
12. Enjoy.

Nutrient Info Per Serving

Calories: 594 | Carbs: 56 g | Fibre: 10 g | Protein: 33 g | Fat: 25 g | Saturated Fat: 11 g

Cheesy Stuffed Peppers

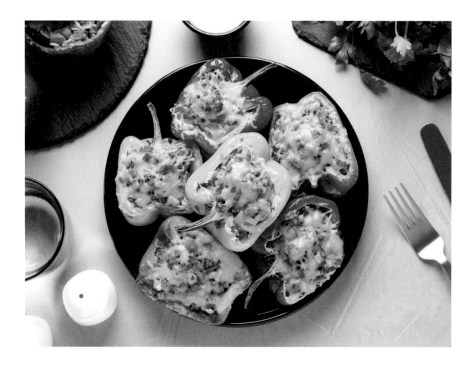

I love stuffed vegetables and peppers are perfect little vegetable bowls!

Servings: 2

Time to make: 15 minutes

Ingredients

- 80 g wholegrain rice, uncooked
- 2 teaspoons of extra virgin olive oil
- 3 cloves of garlic, chopped
- 2 small onions, chopped
- 2 teaspoons of cumin
- 2 teaspoons of coriander (cilantro)
- 200 g beef mince, extra lean (5% fat)
- 2 tablespoons of tomato purée
- Half of a beef stock cube, make 400 mL of stock
- 2 peppers, chopped in half and deseeded
- 40 g cheddar cheese, grated
- Salt and pepper

Instructions

1. Preheat the oven to 180°C / fan 160°C / 350°F / gas mark 4.
2. Boil water in a medium pot and cook the rice for 15 minutes.
3. Heat 1 teaspoon of oil in a frying pan over a medium heat.
4. Add the garlic, onion, and spices and stir for 2 minutes.
5. Add the beef mince, season with salt and pepper and cook until there is no pink left.
6. Add the tomato purée and cook for 30 seconds, stirring all the time.
7. Add half the stock and simmer for 3 minutes.
8. Add the cooked rice and stir well.
9. Arrange the halved peppers in a large oven dish (see picture).
10. Fill the peppers with as much filling as possible (flatten down with the back of a spoon and pile it on!).
11. Add the rest of the stock to the bottom of the dish and cover the dish tightly with tin foil. Cook for 30 minutes.
12. Remove the foil and top each pepper with an even amount of cheese. Put the dish back in for another 5 minutes.
13. Divide between 2 dishes.

Nutrient Info Per Serving

Calories: 508 | Carbs: 48 g | Fibre: 11 g | Protein: 37 g | Fat: 16 g | Saturated Fat: 6 g

Sticky Beef and Asparagus

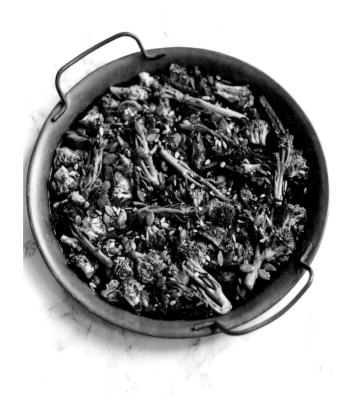

As you know by now, iron is an essential nutrient for female athletes (see chapter 1). This dish contains over half of your daily requirements along with 100% of your vitamin C requirements, which assists with the absorption of iron.

Servings: 2

Time to make: 20 minutes

Ingredients

- 2 teaspoons of extra virgin olive oil
- 200 g lean beef steak, diced
- 1 small red onion, finely diced
- 2 cloves of garlic, chopped
- 2 tablespoons of reduced sodium/light soy sauce
- 1 tablespoon honey
- Half a vegetable stock cube (make 150 mL stock with it)
- 1 head of broccoli (200 g), chopped
- 250 g asparagus, chopped (cut off the bottom 2" and throw away)
- 100 g whole wheat noodles
- 2 teaspoons of sesame seeds
- Half a teaspoon of chilli flakes
- Half a teaspoon of thyme
- Salt and pepper

Instructions

1. Place frying pan over a medium-high heat, add 1 teaspoon of oil and sear the steak until cooked to your liking. Remove steak pieces from the pan and leave to one side.
2. Reduce the heat to medium, add the remaining oil to the same pan, then add the onion and garlic and fry until soft (about 5 minutes).
3. Add soy sauce, honey and vegetable stock, stir until combined.
4. Add the chopped broccoli and asparagus, bring to a boil, stir until sauce has thickened (approximately 5 minutes).
5. Add the beef back into the mixture, mix well and stir fry for another 3 minutes.
6. Cook the noodles to packet instructions.
7. Divide between 2 dishes and top each dish with a teaspoon of sesame seeds.

Nutrient Info Per Serving

Calories: 521 | Carbs: 57 g | Fibre: 10 g | Protein: 40 g | Fat: 13 g | Saturated Fat: 4 g

Quick Quesadillas

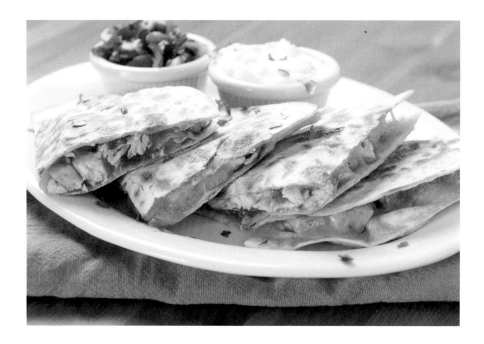

Delicious, nutritious and quick!

Servings: 2

Time to make: 10 minutes

Ingredients

- Half a tin of kidney beans, drained
- 1 teaspoon of fajita seasoning
- 150 g cooked sandwich chicken
- Half a pepper, chopped
- 1 scallion, chopped
- Salt and pepper
- 1 teaspoon of extra virgin olive oil
- 2 tortilla wraps
- 4 tablespoons of salsa dip
- 60 g of grated cheddar cheese

Instructions

1. Drain and add the kidney beans to a bowl, heat for 20 seconds in the microwave.
2. Once heated, mash the beans with the fajita seasoning.
3. Add the chicken, chopped pepper and the scallion to a second bowl and season with salt and pepper.
4. Brush a large frying pan with 1 teaspoon of oil (you can use balled up kitchen paper to do this). The key to a crispy quesadilla is less oil in the pan, not more. Warm the pan over a medium-high heat.
5. Place 1 tortilla wrap in the pan and add 2 tablespoons of salsa, spread out with the back of the spoon, then sprinkle all over with half the cheese.
6. Spread half the chicken and veg filling in a single layer over just half the tortilla. Spreading the filling over only half makes the quesadilla easier to fold.
7. Watch for the cheese to melt. Once the cheese starts to melt, begin lifting a corner of the tortilla with a spatula and check the underside to see if it is browning.
8. When the cheese has completely melted and you see golden brown spots on the underside of the tortilla, the wrap is ready to turn. Use the spatula to fold the quesadilla in half, sandwiching the filling by pressing down on with the back of the spatula.
9. Slide the quesadilla onto a cutting board. Let cool for a minute for the cheese to set, then cut into wedges.
10. Wipe the pan clean if needed, melt another teaspoon of oil and cook the other quesadilla as described.

Nutrient Info Per Serving

Calories: 511 | Carbs: 46 g | Fibre: 9 g | Protein: 37 g | Fat: 18 g | Saturated Fat: 4 g

Supped Up Tuna Melt

Tuna mayo is a standard sandwich filling, and I like to take the classics and boost their nutrient profile. This dish is high in protein, fibre and slow-releasing carbohydrates.

Servings: 2

Time to make: 10 minutes

Ingredients

- 2 large slices of sourdough bread
- 1 tin of tuna, drained
- Half a tin of chickpeas
- 2 handfuls of rocket (arugula), chopped
- 3 tablespoons of sweetcorn
- 1 handful of cherry tomatoes, chopped
- 1 tablespoon of mayonnaise
- Salt and pepper
- 2 slices of cheddar cheese

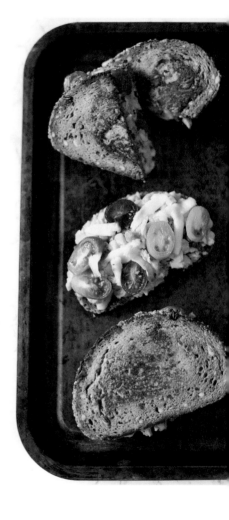

Instructions

1. Toast the sourdough.
2. While the bread is toasting, add the tuna, chickpeas, rocket, sweetcorn, tomatoes and mayonnaise to a bowl.
3. Season with salt and pepper and mix well.
4. Top each piece of toast with half the mix and top with a slice of cheese.
5. Melt the cheese under a grill for a couple of minutes.

Nutrient Info Per Serving

Calories: 487 | Carbs: 53 g | Fibre: 7 g | Protein: 28 g | Fat: 16 g | Saturated Fat: 6 g

Recovery Day Dinners

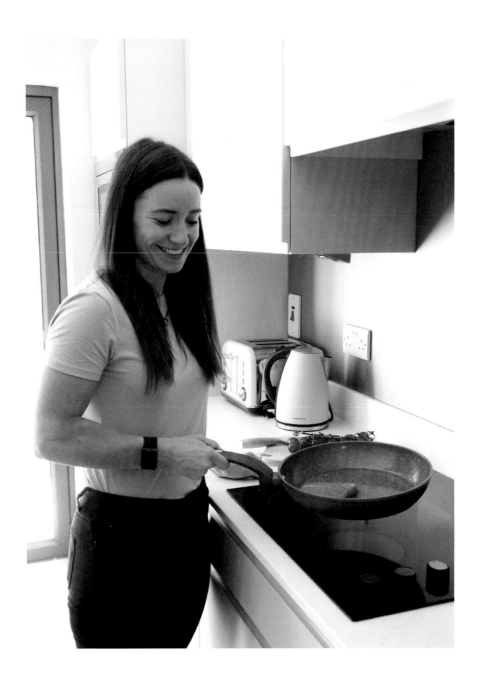

Beef Chow Mein

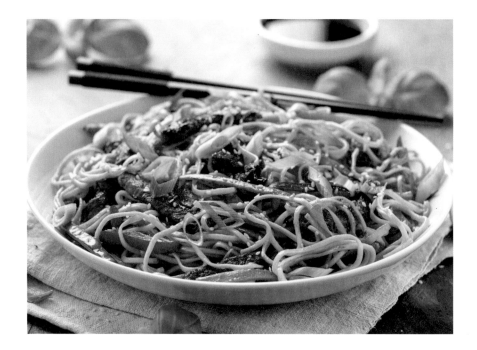

I've already mentioned how important a good condiment cupboard is, and this recipe will encourage you to stock up on any stir fry condiments you don't have!

Servings: 2

Time to make: 30 minutes

Ingredients

- 100 g of whole wheat noodles
- 3 teaspoons of sesame oil
- 160 g lean beef steak, sliced into thin strips
- 2 tablespoons of reduce sodium/light soy sauce
- 2 teaspoons of rice vinegar
- White pepper
- Salt
- 1 garlic clove, finely diced/crushed
- 100 g mangetout

- 150 g baby corn
- 2 handfuls of mushrooms, chopped
- Half a teaspoon of brown sugar
- 1 scallion chopped

Instructions

1. Cook the noodles in a large pan of boiling water according to packet instructions, then drain and place them in cold water. Drain thoroughly, toss them with 1 teaspoon of sesame oil and set aside.
2. Combine beef with 1 tablespoon soy sauce, 1 teaspoon rice vinegar, half a teaspoon sesame oil, quarter of a teaspoon white pepper and quarter of a teaspoon salt, cover and leave to marinate in the fridge for about 30 minutes.
3. Heat a wok over a high heat. Add half a teaspoon of sesame oil and, when it is very hot and slightly smoking, add the beef mix.
4. Stir fry for about 2 minutes and then transfer to a plate.
5. Wipe the wok clean, reheat until it is very hot then add 1 teaspoon of sesame oil.
6. Add the garlic and stir fry for 10 seconds, add chopped mangetout, baby corn and mushrooms, and stir fry for about 1 minute.
7. Add the noodles, 1 tablespoon soy sauce, 1 teaspoon rice vinegar, quarter of a teaspoon of white pepper, quarter of a teaspoon brown sugar, 1 finely chopped scallion and quarter of a teaspoon salt.
8. Stir fry for 2 minutes. Return the beef and any juices to the noodle mixture. Stir fry for about 4 minutes or until the beef is cooked.
9. Add half a teaspoon of sesame oil and give the mixture a final stir.
10. Divide between 2 plates and top with some sesame seeds.

Nutrient Info Per Serving

Calories: 400 | Carbs: 48 g | Fibre: 7 g | Protein: 29 g | Fat: 9 g | Saturated Fat: 2 g

Pan-Fried Salmon and Sweet Potato

This dish packed full of micronutrients, healthy fats and protein. It is an ideal recovery day meal and will help you combat stress that training has placed on your body.

Servings: 2

Time to make: 30 minutes

Ingredients

- 300 g sweet potato, peeled and chopped into small cubes (about 2 × 2")
- 2 teaspoons of extra virgin olive oil
- 2 medium salmon fillets
- Salt and pepper
- 2 tablespoons of natural yogurt
- Half a clove of garlic, finely diced/crushed
- 1 tablespoon of dried dill
- 2 teaspoons of pine nuts
- 2 handfuls of fresh spinach
- 20 g feta cheese, crumbled
- 100 g pickled beetroot, sliced

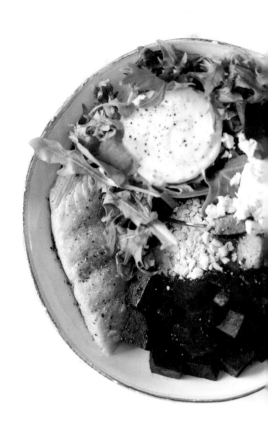

Instructions

1. Boil the sweet potato cubes for 5 minutes.
2. Add 1 teaspoon of extra virgin olive oil to a frying pan over medium heat.
3. Drain the sweet potato, add to the pan and cook for 5 minutes until lightly browned.
4. Remove the and set to one side.
5. Season salmon on both sides with salt and pepper.
6. Add 1 teaspoon of oil to the pan, add salmon fillets skin side up and cook for 4 minutes, turn and cook for 3 minutes.
7. While the salmon is cooking, make yogurt dressing by combining yogurt, garlic, dill, salt and pepper to a bowl and mix well.
8. Toast the pine nuts in a small saucepan for a couple of minutes (careful as they will burn easily).
9. Make salad on each plate by adding half the bag of greens, feta, beetroot and pine nuts.
10. Add the sweet potato and salmon to the plates and top each salmon fillet with half of the yogurt dressing.

Nutrient Info Per Serving

Calories: 601 | Carbs: 38 g | Fibre: 5 g | Protein: 38 g | Fat: 32 g | Saturated Fat: 7 g

Seafood Tagliatelle

This is one of my fancier dishes, so a nice option if you have friends over for dinner or if you ever have to cook for your teammates!

Serves: 4

Time to make: 40 minutes

Ingredients

- 2 tablespoons of butter
- 170 g peeled and cooked prawns (shrimp)
- 250 g seafood mix
- Salt and pepper
- 1 small onion, diced
- 3 cloves of garlic, finely chopped/diced
- 180 mL milk
- Half of a chicken stock cube, make 180 mL of stock
- 40 g Parmesan cheese, grated
- 400 g tomatoes, diced
- 200 g broccoli, chopped
- 250 g asparagus, halved
- 1 small handful of fresh parsley, chopped
- Half a lemon, juiced
- 450 g fresh tagliatelle pasta

Instructions

1. In a large pan over medium heat, melt 1 tablespoon butter.
2. Add prawns and seafood mix and season with salt and pepper. Cook 2 minutes per side, then transfer to a plate.
3. Add the onion and garlic and cook until soft and fragrant, about 3 minutes.
4. Add milk, stock, half the parmesan, tomatoes, broccoli, asparagus, parsley.
5. Season with salt and pepper, bring to the boil and then reduce the heat to low/medium.

6. Simmer 5 minutes more, then return the seafood mix and toss until combined. Squeeze in the lemon juice and simmer while the pasta cooks.
7. In a large pot of salted boiling water, cook tagliatelle according to package directions until al dente (about 4 minutes). Drain and return to the pot.
8. Add cooked tagliatelle to the seafood mix and toss until fully coated.
9. Divide between 4 plates. Garnish with parsley and sprinkle with the rest of the parmesan.

Nutrient Info Per Serving

Calories: 468 | Carbs: 41 g | Fibre: 7g | Protein: 37 g | Fat: 16 g | Saturated Fat: 7 g

Chicken and Cashew Stir Fry

On recovery days we should aim to increase our healthy fats and adding nuts to our main meals can help us to do that. Cashews go well in stir fries, but you can add whatever nuts or seeds you prefer!

Serves: 2

Time to make: 20 minutes

Ingredients

- 1 lemon
- Quarter of a vegetable stock cube (make 50 mL stock)
- 1 tablespoon of honey
- 1 tablespoon of reduced sodium/ light soy sauce
- 1 teaspoon of extra virgin olive oil
- 200 g chicken breast, diced
- Large handful of mushrooms, chopped
- 25 g cashew nuts
- 1 large carrot, sliced diagonally
- 100 g mangetout
- 100 g baby sweetcorn
- 2 cloves of garlic, chopped
- 2 scallions, chopped
- 200 g wholemeal noodles
- Salt and pepper

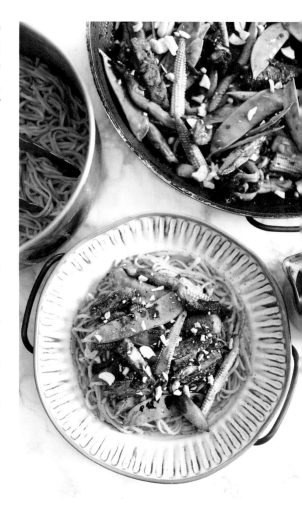

Instructions

1. Grate some lemon zest into a bowl and set aside.
2. Juice the lemon and whisk 3 tbsp of the juice with 50 mL stock, honey and soy sauce in a small bowl.
3. Heat the oil in a large frying pan over medium-high heat.
4. Add diced chicken pieces, season with salt and pepper, and fry until cooked through.
5. Transfer to a plate with tongs.
6. Add mushrooms, cashews and carrots to the pan and cook until the carrots are just tender, about 5 minutes.
7. Add the rest of the vegetables, garlic and the reserved lemon zest.
8. Cook, stirring, for about 30 seconds.
9. Whisk the stock mixture and add to the pan.
10. Cook, stirring for 2–3 minutes.
11. Add scallion greens and the chicken and any accumulated juices. Cook, stirring, until heated through, 1–2 minutes.
12. Cook noodles according to packet instructions.
13. Divide stir fry and noodles between 2 plates.

Nutrient Info Per Serving

Calories: 477 | Carbs: 60 g | Fibre: 10 g | Protein: 37 g | Fat: 10 g | Saturated Fat: 2 g

Chicken and Mushroom Stroganoff

Traditional stroganoff uses sour cream, and if you are looking to increase your calorie intake on recovery day, you can swap the yogurt for sour cream if you wish.

Serves: 2

Time to make: 20 minutes

Ingredients

- 1 teaspoon of butter
- 1 onion, diced
- 3 cloves of garlic, chopped
- 200 g chicken breast, diced
- 200 g mushrooms, chopped
- Salt and pepper
- Quarter of a vegetable stock cube (make 100 mL stock)
- 1 pepper, chopped
- Half a teaspoon of dried dill
- 150 g natural yogurt
- 250 g packet of microwave rice

Instructions

1. Place the frying pan over medium heat, add butter, onion and garlic to the pan and cook for 5 minutes until softened and fragrant.
2. Add the chicken and mushrooms to the same pan, turn up the heat to medium-high, and cook until chicken pieces are no longer pink on the outside, season with salt and pepper.
3. Add stock and simmer for 5 minutes.
4. Add the chopped pepper and dill and cook for 3 minutes.

5. Remove pan from heat and allow to cool for 5–10 minutes.
6. Add yogurt to pan and stir until combined well. If you add the yogurt while the pan is still hot, it may split – it will taste just as nice, only it will look a little strange!
7. While the pan is cooling, microwave the rice according to the packet instructions.
8. Divide the rice and the stroganoff between 2 dishes.

Nutrient Info Per Serving

Calories: 462 | Carbs: 54 g | Fibre: 6 g | Protein: 36 g | Fat: 11 g | Saturated Fat: 5 g

Prawn and Chorizo Jambalaya

One-pot recipes are ideal for meal prep. The key to meal prep is to find a handful of recipes you are happy to eat repeatedly, and this dish is so tasty it's one my clients request over and over!

Serves: 4

Time to make: 30 minutes

Ingredients

- 300 g cooked and peeled prawns (shrimp)
- 1 tablespoon extra virgin olive oil
- 1 onion, diced
- 1 pepper, chopped
- 3 cloves of garlic, chopped
- 75 g chorizo, chopped
- 1 tablespoon of Cajun spice mix
- 1 tin of chopped tomatoes
- Half a vegetable stock cube (make 350 mL of stock)
- 250 g long grain rice, uncooked
- 200 g frozen peas
- Salt and pepper

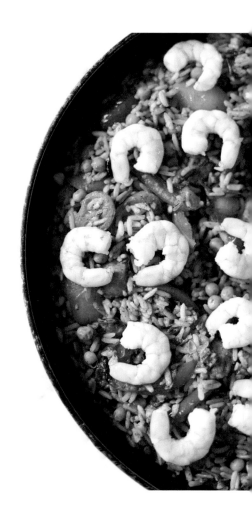

Instructions

1. If you are using frozen prawns, take them out the night before and defrost in the fridge overnight.
2. Heat the oil in a large frying pan (with a lid) over a medium-high heat.
3. Add in the diced onion, and cook for 3-4 minutes until soft.
4. Add the chopped pepper, garlic, chorizo, salt and pepper, and Cajun seasoning, and cook for 5 minutes more.
5. Add the tin of tomatoes and 350 mL vegetable stock. Then add in the long grain rice and stir well.
6. Bring to the boil and then reduce to a simmer.
7. Cover with the lid and simmer for 15–20 minutes until the rice is tender, check regularly and stir well every 5 minutes, if the mix starts to dry out quickly then reduce the heat slightly.
8. Add in the peas and cooked prawns for the last 5 minute of the cooking time.
9. Divide between four dishes, and enjoy!

Nutrient Info Per Serving

Calories: 468 | Carbs: 63 g | Fibre: 6 g | Protein: 25 g | Fat: 11 g | Saturated Fat: 5 g

Roast Red Pepper Pasta

The pasta sauce for this dish is made from roast red peppers and low-fat cottage cheese. This makes it a far more nutritious option compared with shop-bought pasta sauce jars.

Serves: 4

Time to make: 40 minutes

Ingredients

- 2 teaspoons of extra virgin olive oil
- 4 cloves of garlic, finely chopped
- 1 onion, diced
- 1 tablespoon of dried mixed herbs
- Salt and pepper
- Jar of roasted red peppers (approx. 320 g jar)
- 250 g plain fat-free cottage cheese
- 2 medium chicken breasts, diced
- Handful of mushrooms, chopped
- 1 pepper, chopped
- 300 g fresh pasta (any kind you want)
- Handful of cherry tomatoes

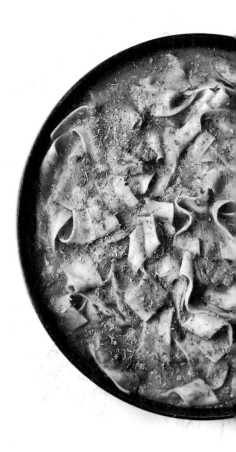

Instructions

1. Heat 1 teaspoon of the oil in a pan over low–medium heat.
2. Add the garlic and onion and cook for a couple of minutes until soft.
3. Add the mixed herbs, salt and pepper and cook for about 3 minutes, stirring constantly.
4. Add the jar of red peppers to a blender/food processor and blend.
5. Add the contents of the pan to the processor and blend.
6. Add the quark, blend and set aside your pasta sauce.
7. In the pan heat the second teaspoon of oil.
8. Add the chicken and mushrooms and cook for about 5–7 minutes until the chicken is nearly cooked.
9. Add the chopped peppers and cook while stirring for about 3 minutes.
10. While the chicken and veg are cooking, boil water in a large saucepan and cook the pasta (fresh pasta only take 3–4 minutes to cook).
11. Add the pasta sauce to the pan with the chicken and veg and heat through.
12. Divide the pasta and the pasta sauce mix evenly between four dishes.

Nutrient Info Per Serving

Calories: 434 | Carbs: 56 g | Fibre: 7 g | Protein: 34 g | Fat: 7 g | Saturated Fat: 2 g

Mexican Lasagne

I love getting creative when creating new recipes. This recipe takes the layering concept of a traditional lasagne and uses some not-so-traditional ingredients!

Serves: 6

Time to make: 45 minutes

Ingredients

- 2 tablespoons of extra virgin olive oil
- 4 cloves of garlic, finely chopped
- 1 medium red onion, finely chopped
- 2 peppers, chopped
- 35 g fajita seasoning
- 400 g chicken breast, diced
- 2 tins of chopped tomatoes
- 2 small tins of sweetcorn, drained
- 1 tin of mixed beans, drained
- 170 g cheddar cheese, grated
- 4 wholemeal tortilla wraps
- 1 packet of microwavable wholegrain rice (250 g)
- Salt and pepper

Instructions

1. Preheat the oven to 180°C / fan 160°C / 350°F / gas mark 4.
2. Heat 1 tablespoon of oil in a large pan over medium heat.
3. Add the garlic, onion and peppers and fry for a few minutes until soft.
4. Add half of the packet of seasoning and stir fry for a couple of minutes, then remove the veg from the pan and set to one side.
5. Add the other tablespoon of oil to the pan and add the chicken. Stir fry until the chicken is browned, then add the rest of the seasoning.
6. Add the tins of tomatoes to the pan and simmer for 5 minutes.

7. Add the sweetcorn and the mixed beans and simmer for 5 minutes.
8. Add half the chicken and bean mix to a large oven dish, then half of the veg mix and top with 70 g cheese.
9. Cut 2 large wraps in half and arrange them in the dish with the flat side along the edge.
10. Then top with the rest of the pan mix, then the veg mix.
11. Cut the other 2 wraps in half and place on top of the dish.
12. Top the wraps with the rest of the cheese.
13. Pop the dish into the oven for 10 minutes.
14. Divide into six portions.

Nutrient Info Per Serving

Calories: 555 | Carbs: 56 g | Protein: 37 g | Fat: 21 g | Fibre: 9 g

All the Spuds Fish Pie

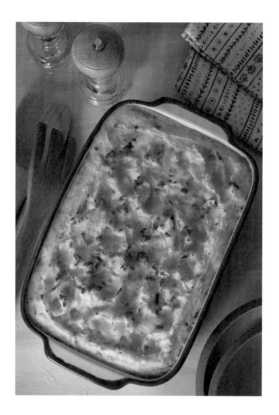

This is nutrient-dense comfort food. It is packed full of vitamins, minerals, protein and healthy fats – an ideal recovery day dinner, especially on those cold winter evenings!

Serves: 4

Time to make: 45 minutes

Ingredients

- 400 g white potatoes
- 1 medium sweet potato
- 2 tablespoons of butter
- 1 medium onion, finely chopped
- 150 g mushrooms, chopped

- Half a teaspoon of garlic powder
- 2 teaspoons of dried mixed herbs
- 1 large carrot, peeled and chopped
- Salt and pepper
- 500 g seafood mix
- Splash of milk
- 250 mL cooking cream
- 1 head of broccoli, chopped to small pieces
- 100 g frozen peas
- 60 g cheddar cheese, grated

Instructions

1. Preheat the oven to oven to 180°C / fan 160°C / 350°F / gas mark 4.
2. Chop the potatoes into cubes and boil in salted water (I leave the skins on but it's up to you!)
3. While potatoes are cooking, heat 1 tablespoon of butter in a large saucepan over a medium heat.
4. Add the onion and cook for a couple of minutes until soft, then add the mushrooms and cook for 5 minutes.
5. Add the garlic and mixed herbs, cook for another couple of minutes.
6. Add the carrot and season with salt and pepper.
7. Add the mixed seafood, cook for about 3 minutes and then add the cooking cream, mix well.
8. When the potatoes are done, season well with salt and pepper, add a tablespoon of butter and a splash of milk. Mash well.
9. Add broccoli and peas to the seafood pan and cook for about 3 minutes.
10. Add the seafood mix to a baking dish and top with the mash, sprinkle the cheese over the top.
11. Pop in the oven for 15 minutes until the top turn slightly brown.
12. Aim to get about four portions from it.

Nutrient Info Per Serving

Calories: 602 | Carbs: 44 g | Protein: 37 g | Fat: 29 g | Fibre: 10 g

Pesto Salmon and Roast Veg

One-tray recipes are ideal for a quick, no fuss meal with minimal clean up! Nutritious dishes don't have to be complex, simple can work just as well with the right ingredients.

Serves: 2

Time to make: 40 minutes

Ingredients

- 200 g baby potatoes, sliced
- 1 parsnip, peeled and sliced
- 2 carrots, peeled and sliced
- 1 teaspoon extra virgin olive oil
- 2 teaspoons of dried rosemary
- Salt and pepper
- 2 teaspoons of basil pesto
- 2 salmon fillets
- 80 g mozzarella
- Handful of cherry tomatoes, halved
- 4 cloves of garlic, chopped
- 1 teaspoon of garlic powder

Instructions

1. Preheat the oven to 220°C / fan 200°C / 425°F / gas mark 7.
2. Add the sliced potatoes and chopped vegetables to a large oven dish.
3. Drizzle with oil and season well with rosemary, salt and pepper.
4. Put the dish in the oven for 10 minutes.
5. Add 1 teaspoon of basil pesto on top of each salmon fillet.
6. Arrange the mozzarella and tomatoes over the top as in the picture.
7. After 10 minutes remove the oven dish, turn the veg and then place the salmon fillets on top.
8. Place back in the oven for 13–15 minutes.
9. Divide between two dishes.

Nutrient Info Per Serving

Calories: 546 | Carbs: 32 g | Protein: 37 g | Fat: 27 g | Fibre: 9 g

Chapter 10

High Nutrient Treats

I love making high nutrient treats and will usually try and include a batch a week in my meal prep. Here are 10 of my favourites, and you can find lots more on my Instagram page @bridgenutrition. Some of them have flavoured protein powder to help you hit your daily targets and to add a little sweetness! You can choose any type you like but I recommend whey or casein protein.

Just as you would have done for the training day and recovery day recipes, it's a good idea to plan out what high nutrient treats you wish try to make shopping and meal prep easier. A great way to start is making a list of the top five treats you want to try first.

Bridge Nutrition PB Protein Bars

Makes 10 bars

Time to make: 20 minutes

Ingredients

- 120 g peanut butter, no added sugar/ palm oil
- 1 teaspoon vanilla essence
- 100 g honey
- 120 g oats
- 50 g chocolate
- 100 g protein powder (chocolate/ vanilla flavour)

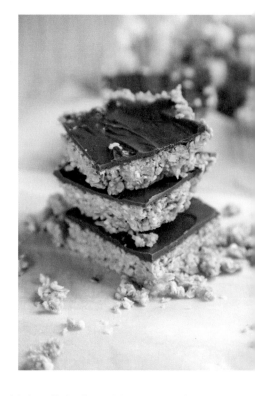

Instructions

1. Heat the peanut butter, vanilla extract and honey in a small saucepan over a medium heat until they have melted, mix well.
2. Add all the dry ingredients to a large bowl and mix well.
3. Add in the melted mix and combine well. If it is a little dry, add a couple of tablespoons of water (you need it wet enough to make a dough).
4. Line a baking tray with greaseproof paper and press the mix in firmly with clean hands.
5. Chill for a couple of hours in the freezer.
6. When chilled, melt the chocolate in the microwave (do this in 30-second intervals as chocolate can easily burn).
7. Drizzle over the top of the baking try and chill for another 20 minutes.
8. Cut into 10 bars.
9. Store in an airtight container in the fridge for up to a week or in the freezer for up to a month.

Nutrient Info (per bar)

Calories: 231 | Carbs: 20 g | Fibre: 2 g | Protein: 12 g | Fat: 11 g | Saturated Fat: 3 g

Granola Bars

Makes 12 bars

Time to make: 20 minutes

Ingredients

- 65 g peanut butter (no added salt/sugar)
- 4 tablespoons of honey
- 130 g mixed nuts, chopped
- 140 g oats
- 1 teaspoon Vanilla essence
- 50 g chocolate chips

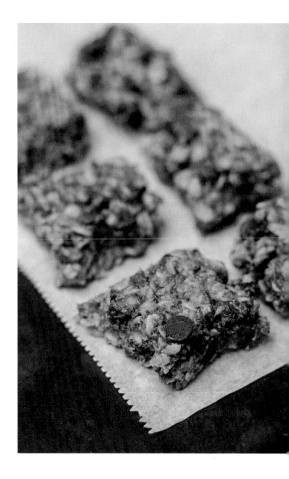

Instructions

1. Melt the peanut butter and honey in a small bowl over a medium heat.
2. Roughly chop the nuts and add to a bowl with the rest of the dry ingredients.
3. Add the honey/peanut butter, mix well, if the mix is a little dry add a couple of tablespoons of water.
4. Line a small baking dish with greaseproof paper.
5. Add the mix and press down firmly with a spoon.
6. Pop in the fridge overnight.
7. Cut into 12 bars.
8. Store in an airtight container in the fridge for up to a week or in the freezer for up to a month.

Nutrient Info (per bar)

Calories: 201 | Carbs: 17 g | Fibre: 2 g | Protein: 5 g | Fat: 12 g | Saturated Fat: 2 g

Recovery Bars

Makes 10 bars

Time to make: 25 minutes

Ingredients

- 8 pitted dates
- 180 g oats
- 80 g protein powder (chocolate/vanilla flavour)
- 25 g cocoa powder
- 150 mL milk
- Pinch of salt
- 1 teaspoon vanilla essence
- 60 g 80%+ dark chocolate

Instructions

1. Soak the dates in a bowl of boiling water for 5 minutes, then roughly chop.
2. In a food processor, blend the oats into a flour, add the protein and the dates and blend until the dates are broken into tiny pieces almost not visible (the mix will have turned to a brown-ish flour colour).
3. Add the cocoa powder, milk, salt and vanilla and blend into a thick heavy dough.
4. Spoon the mix into a lined bread tin, press to compact and smooth out over the top.
5. Melt the chocolate in the microwave for 30-second intervals (it will burn easily, so be careful).
6. Drizzle over with the melted chocolate.
7. Place in the freezer (15–20 minutes) or fridge for 45 minutes to set.
8. Tip when cutting into bars, heat the knife so it slides through the hardened chocolate topping without cracking it.
9. Store in an airtight container in the fridge for up to a week or in the freezer for up to a month.

Nutrient Info (per bar)

Calories: 214 | Carbs: 30 g | Fibre: 4 g | Protein: 10 g | Fat: 5 g | Saturated Fat: 2 g

Chocolate Chia Cookies

Makes 10 cookies

Time to make: 35 minutes

Ingredients

- 2 bananas
- 120 mL skimmed milk
- 100 g oats
- 50 g chocolate chips
- 50 g protein powder (chocolate or vanilla)
- 3 teaspoons of cocoa powder
- 1 tablespoon of chia seeds
- 1 teaspoon of baking powder

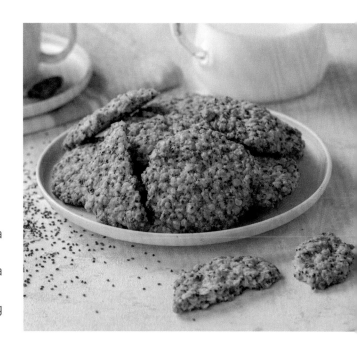

Instructions

1. Preheat the oven to 180°C / fan 160°C / 350°F / gas mark 4.
2. Mash the bananas in a bowl and add the rest of the ingredients, mix well.
3. Line a baking tray with greaseproof paper.
4. With a wet spoon, spoon out 10 even amounts of the mixture.
5. Wet your fingers and smooth the mounds into cookie shapes.
6. Bake for 25 minutes.
7. Store in an airtight container in the fridge for up to a week or in the freezer for up to a month.

Nutrient Info (per bar)

Calories: 120 | Carbs: 14 g | Fibre: 2 g | Protein: 7 g | Fat: 4 g | Saturated Fat: 2 g

Protein Peanut Butter Cups

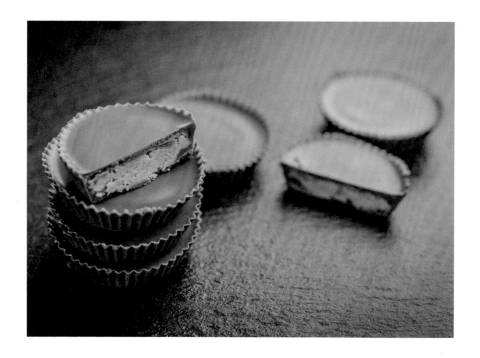

Makes 12 cups

Time to make: 45 minutes

Ingredients

- 200 g dark chocolate
- 150 mL skimmed milk
- 2 scoops of chocolate protein powder
- 100 g peanut butter (no palm oil/sugar)
- 1 scoop of vanilla protein powder

Instructions

1. Add 100 g dark chocolate to a jug/bowl and add 50 mL of low-fat milk.
2. Heat for 30 seconds in a microwave, take out and stir well until all the chocolate has melted.
3. Add 1 scoop of chocolate protein powder and stir until well mixed.
4. Add bun casings to a muffin tray, add 1 or 2 teaspoons of chocolate mix to each casing and spread to cover the bottom.
5. Pop into the freezer for 15 minutes.
6. Add the peanut butter to a jug/bowl and heat for 30 seconds in a microwave, take out and stir well.
7. Add 1 scoop of vanilla protein powder and stir until well mixed.
8. Add 1 teaspoon of peanut butter mix to each casing and spread it so it's even.
9. Pop back into the freezer for 15 minutes.
10. Add 100 g of dark chocolate to a jug/bowl and add 100 mL low-fat milk.
11. Heat for 30 seconds in a microwave, take out and stir well until all the chocolate has melted.
12. Add 1 scoop of chocolate protein powder and stir until well mixed.
13. Add 1or 2 teaspoons of chocolate mix to each casing and spread it until it covers the peanut butter.
14. Pop back into the freezer for 2 hours to set.
15. Store in an airtight container in the fridge or the freezer.

Nutrient Info (per bar)

Calories: 183 | **Carbs: 7 g** | **Fibre: 3 g** | **Protein: 10 g** | **Fat: 12 g** | **Saturated Fat: 6 g**

Crispy Quinoa Bars

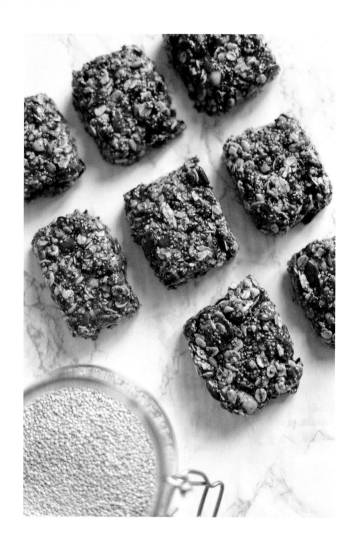

Makes 12 bars

Time to make: 40 minutes

Ingredients

- 150 g quinoa
- 80 g porridge oats (oatmeal)
- 3 tablespoons pumpkin seeds
- 3 tablespoons sunflower seeds
- 3 tablespoons chia seeds
- 3 tablespoons blueberries, dried
- 60 g 80% dark chocolate
- 170 g cashew nut butter
- 150 g honey

Instructions

1. Rinse the quinoa well (in a flour sieve) and then add it to a large baking dish.
2. Pop it in the oven at oven to 180°C / fan 160°C / 350°F / gas mark 4 for 10 minutes until it has dried.
3. Add it to a large pan over medium to high heat until it starts to brown, and you hear a popping (kind of like popcorn).
4. Be careful not to let it burn, you want it only slightly browned.
5. Add the quinoa to a large bowl with the porridge, seeds, dried blueberries and chocolate.
6. In a small saucepan, melt the cashew nut butter and honey over a medium heat. Stir all the time until it melts.
7. Add this to the dry mix and work together until well mixed.
8. Line a baking dish with cling film and add in the mix.
9. Wet your hands and press it into the dish, smooth off the edges and the top.
10. Pop into the freezer for at least an hour.
11. Cut into 12 bars.
12. Store in an airtight container for up to a week in the fridge or a month in the freezer.

Nutrient Info (per bar)

Calories: 265 | Carbs: 28 g | Fibre: 4 g | Protein: 6 g | Fat: 14 g | Saturated Fat: 3 g

Fuelling Flapjacks

Makes 10 flapjacks

Time to make: 30 minutes

Ingredients

- 80 g butter
- 100 g maple syrup
- 100 mL skimmed milk
- 250 g oats
- 50 g raisins
- 60 g protein powder (chocolate or vanilla)

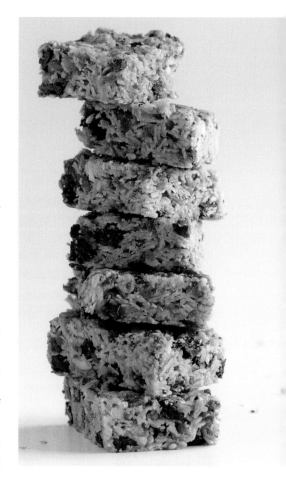

Instructions

1. Preheat the oven to 180°C / fan 160°C / 350°F / gas mark 4.
2. Melt the butter, maple syrup and milk in a large saucepan over low heat.
3. When the butter is melted, add the rest of the ingredients and mix well.
4. Line a baking dish with greaseproof paper.
5. Add the mix to a baking dish. Press it down as much as you can to compact it.
6. Add to the oven and bake for 15–20 minutes (it should be browned on top).
7. Remove from oven, and cut into 10 bars but don't take out of the baking dish.
8. Allow the dish to cool completely before removing the bars.
9. Flapjacks can be stored in an airtight container for up to a week.

Nutrient Info (per bar)

Calories: 228 | Carbs: 27 g | Fibre: 2 g | Protein: 8 g | Fat: 9 g | Saturated Fat: 5 g

Baked Almond Butter Bars

Makes 12 bars

Time to make: 40 minutes

Ingredients

- 170 g almond butter
- 100 g honey
- 150 g oats
- 150 g mixed nuts
- 100 g blueberries, dried
- 100 g cranberries, dried
- 50 g chocolate chips

Instructions

1. Preheat the oven to 160°C / fan 140°C / 325°F / gas mark 3.
2. Heat the almond butter and honey in a small pan, and stir until melted.
3. Add all the dry ingredients, except the chocolate chips, to a bowl and mix.
4. Add the honey/nut butter mix to the dry ingredients and mix well.
5. Press the mix into a non-stick (or line it with greaseproof paper) oven dish well (to whatever thickness you like).
6. Sprinkle the chocolate chips over the top and press in.
7. Pop it into the oven for at least 15–20 minutes (keep an eye that it doesn't burn).
8. Let cool completely, and cut into 12 bars, roughly the same size.
9. Store in the fridge for up to a week, or the freezer for up to a month.

Nutrient Info (per bar)

Calories: 292 | Carbs: 25 g | Fibre: 5 g | Protein: 7 g | Fat: 17 g | Saturated Fat: 3 g

High Protein Brownies

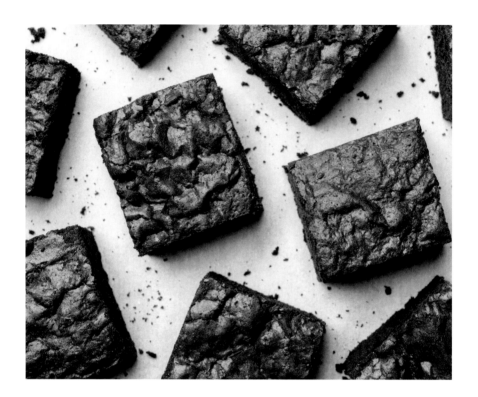

Makes 8 brownies

Time to make: 35 minutes

Ingredients

- 3 tablespoons of oats
- 30 g butter
- 50 g dark chocolate
- 2 eggs
- 150 g 0% Greek yogurt
- 1 tablespoon of honey
- 30 g cocoa powder
- 2 scoops of protein powder (chocolate)
- 200 mL skimmed milk
- 1 teaspoon of baking powder

Instructions

1. Preheat the oven to 180°C / fan 160°C / 350°F / gas mark 4.
2. Add the oats to a food processor and blitz until it's a coarse powder, set aside.
3. Add the butter and the dark chocolate to a bowl, microwave for 10-second intervals stirring as it melts. It will burn easily, so only do it in short intervals.
4. Add the eggs to a large bowl and whisk, add the yogurt and whisk again.
5. Add melted chocolate and honey and whisk until smooth.
6. Sieve in the cocoa powder and protein powder, stir well.
7. Add half the milk, stir. Then add the blitzed oats and baking powder and mix well.
8. Add the rest of the milk, and stir until you have a smooth batter.
9. Line a medium-sized baking tin with greaseproof paper.
10. Pour the batter in, spread so it is even and give it a little shake to smooth out the top.
11. Bake for 25 minutes, then take the mix out with the parchment paper and let it cool completely.
12. Cut into 8 brownies and use a spatula to lift them off the greaseproof paper.
13. Store in an airtight container in the fridge for up to a week, although I doubt they will last that long!

Nutrient Info (per bar)

Calories: 170 | Carbs: 9 g | Fibre: 2 g | Protein: 12 g | Fat: 9 g | Saturated Fat: 5 g

Peanut Butter Protein Brownies

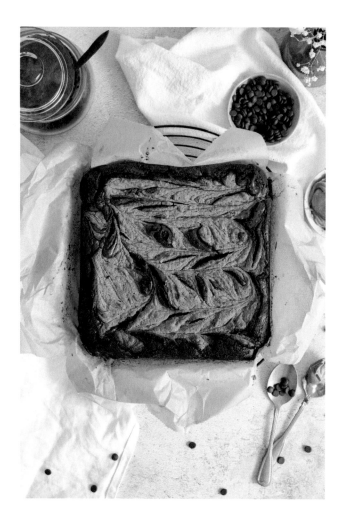

Makes 9 brownies

Time to make: 40 minutes

Ingredients

- 100 g dark chocolate
- 2 teaspoons of coconut oil
- 2 eggs
- 100 mL skimmed milk
- 70 g whole wheat flour
- 1 teaspoon of baking powder
- 2 scoops of protein powder (chocolate)
- Half a teaspoon of salt
- 100 g peanut butter
- 100 g honey
- 1 teaspoon vanilla extract
- 30 g cocoa powder
- 3 tablespoons of oats

Instructions

1. Place chocolate and coconut oil in a medium-sized microwave-safe bowl.
2. Microwave on high for 15-second intervals, stirring in between until chocolate is melted.
3. Let cool.
4. Preheat the oven to 180°C / fan 160°C / 350°F / gas mark 4.
5. Add eggs and milk, mix until combined.
6. Add flour, baking powder, protein powder and a good pinch of salt. Mix until combined.
7. Pour brownie batter into a greased, parchment lined, 8 by 8" (20 by 20 cm) baking pan, making sure that the parchment is overlapping the pan.
8. In a small mixing bowl, combine peanut butter, honey, vanilla extract and a good pinch of salt. Mix until combined. Set aside.
9. Pour peanut butter mixture in several stripes across the top of the brownie batter.
10. With a knife, swirl the peanut butter mixture into the brownie batter.
11. Bake for 15–20 minutes.
12. Let cool before cutting into 9 squares.
13. Enjoy!

Nutrient Info (per bar)

Calories: 273 | Carbs: 20 g | Fibre: 3 g | Protein: 12 g | Fat: 15 g | Saturated Fat: 7 g

Chapter 11

Smoothie Recipes

Fuelling Smoothies

With high carbohydrate requirements on training and game days, players can often struggle to eat the required amount of food, and this is where high carb smoothies are a useful tool for assisted fuelling! The following smoothie recipes are all around 100 g of carbs, which will help you reach your fuelling requirements. If your smoothie is too thick, just add some water and blitz again.

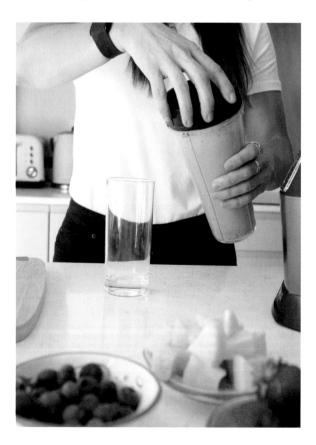

Honey Pear Fuel

Serves: 1

Ingredients

- 1 banana
- 1 pear
- 3 tablespoons of high protein yogurt
- 300 mL orange juice
- 3 tablespoons of honey
- 3 ice cubes

Instruction

1. Add everything to a smoothie maker/blender and blitz!

Nutrient Info Per Serving

Calories: 538 | **Carbs: 111 g** | **Protein: 17 g** | **Fat: 1 g** | **Fibre: 6 g**

Berry Fuel

Serves: 1

Ingredients

- 1 apple
- 100 g frozen mixed berries
- 500 mL dairy milk
- 2 tablespoons of honey
- 3 ice cubes

Instruction

1. Add everything to a smoothie maker/blender and blitz!

Nutrient Info Per Serving

Calories: 542 | **Carbs: 92 g** |
Protein: 19 g | **Fat: 10 g** | **Fibre: 5 g**

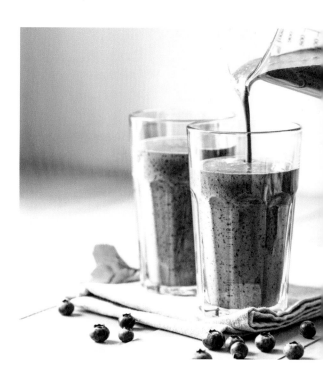

Banana and Yogurt Fuel

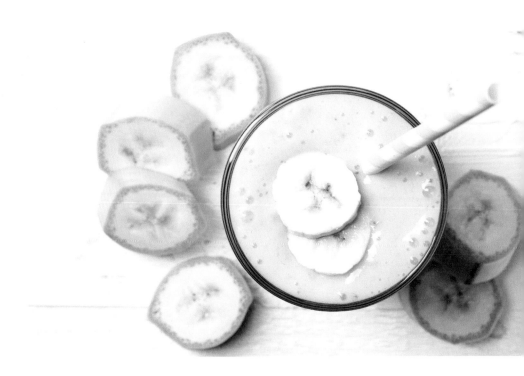

Serves: 1

Ingredients

- 2 bananas
- 300 mL dairy milk
- 2 tablespoons of honey
- 2.5 tablespoons of high protein yogurt
- 3 ice cubes

Instruction

1. Add everything to a smoothie maker/blender and blitz!

Nutrient Info Per Serving

Calories: 532 | Carbs: 98 g | Protein: 21 g | Fat: 5 g | Fibre: 3 g

Mango Fuel

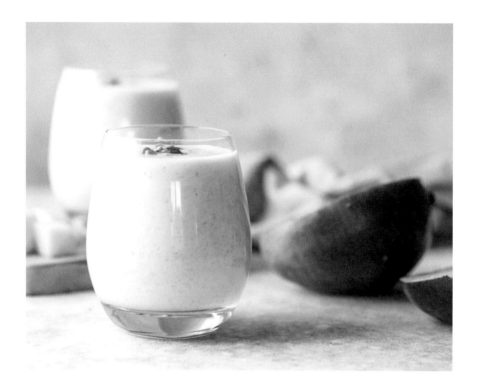

Serves: 1

Ingredients

- 1 banana
- 300 mL dairy milk
- 2 tablespoons of honey
- 125 g frozen mango
- 3 ice cubes

Instruction

1. Add everything to a smoothie maker/blender and blitz!

Nutrient Info Per Serving

Calories: 438 | **Carbs:** 95 g | **Protein:** 14 g | **Fat:** 4 g | **Fibre:** 4 g

Pineapple Fuel

Serves: 1

Ingredients

- 1 apple
- 300 mL orange juice
- 2 tablespoons of honey
- 100 g frozen pineapple
- 1 scoop vanilla protein powder
- 3 ice cubes

Instruction

1. Add everything to a smoothie maker/blender and blitz!

Nutrient Info Per Serving

Calories: 525 | Carbs: 92 g | Protein: 27 g | Fat: 4 g | Fibre: 4 g

Recovery Smoothies

After high-intensity exercise, you may struggle to get in the recommended recovery foods due to a lack of appetite or even nausea. I see this happen quite often with my players, and I find that smoothies can be a great recovery option if an athlete is struggling to eat solid food. Recovery smoothies are already great for an extra dose of nutrients on the go!

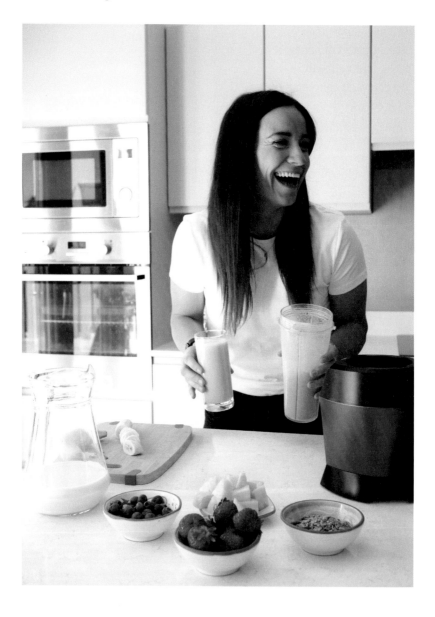

Strawberry Choc

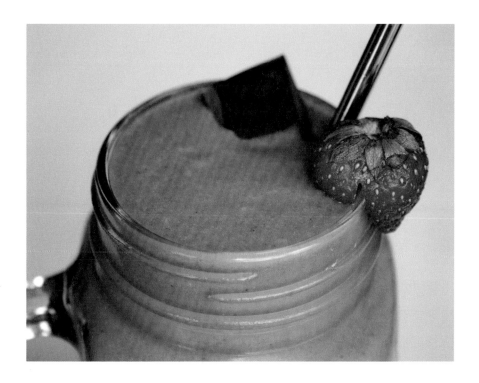

Serves: 1

Ingredients

- 400 mL dairy milk
- 2 tablespoons natural yogurt
- 100 g frozen strawberries
- 1 heaped teaspoon of chocolate spread
- 3 ice cubes

Instruction

1. Add everything to a smoothie maker/blender and blitz!

Nutrient Info Per Serving

Calories: 404 | Carbs: 43 g | Protein: 20 g | Fat: 16 g | Fibre: 3 g

Overnight Muscle Builder

Serves: 1

Ingredients

- 1 banana
- 1 scoop casein protein powder
- 250 mL dairy milk
- 2 tablespoons milled flaxseed
- 3 ice cubes

Instruction

1. Add everything to a smoothie maker/blender and blitz!

Nutrient Info Per Serving

Calories: 355 | Carbs: 33 g | Protein: 30 g | Fat: 10 g | Fibre: 5 g

Fruitie Smoothie

Serves: 1

Ingredients

- 200 mL dairy milk
- 200 g natural yogurt
- 1 apple
- 1 pear
- 1 tablespoon of chia seeds
- 3 ice cubes

Instructions

1. Add everything to a smoothie maker/blender and blitz!

Nutrient Info Per Serving

Calories: 444 | Carbs: 60 g | Protein: 33 g | Fat: 6 g | Fibre: 10 g

Choc Malt Shake

Serves: 1

Ingredients

- 300 mL chocolate milk
- 8 frozen strawberries
- 1 tablespoon of Horlicks powder (or any malt drinking powder)
- 2 tablespoons of oats
- 2 teaspoons of chia seeds
- 3 ice cubes

Instruction

1. Add everything to a smoothie maker/blender and blitz!

Nutrient Info Per Serving

Calories: 453 | Carbs: 69 g | Protein: 20 g | Fat: 9 g | Fibre: 7 g

Super Booster Smoothie

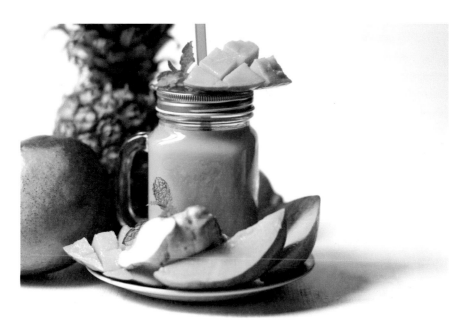

Serves: 1

Ingredients

- 400 mL sparkling water
- 100 g frozen mango
- 100 g frozen pineapple
- 1 banana
- 1 orange
- 1 scoop vanilla protein powder
- 1 lime, juiced
- 3 sprigs of fresh mint
- Half an inch of fresh ginger, peeled
- 3 ice cubes

Instruction

1. Add everything to a smoothie maker/blender and blitz!

Nutrient Info Per Serving

Calories: 438 | Carbs: 66 g | Protein: 28 g | Fat: 4 g | Fibre: 8 g

References

Brown, Natalie et al. "Elite female athletes' experiences and perceptions of the menstrual cycle on training and sport performance." *Scandinavian journal of medicine & science in sports* vol. 31,1 (2021): 52–69. doi:10.1111/sms.13818.

Herzberg, Simone D et al. "The Effect of Menstrual Cycle and Contraceptives on ACL Injuries and Laxity: A Systematic Review and Meta-analysis." *Orthopaedic journal of sports medicine* vol. 5,7 2325967117718781. 21 Jul. 2017, doi:10.1177/2325967117718781.

Lew, Lindsay A et al. "Examination of Sex-Specific Participant Inclusion in Exercise Physiology Endothelial Function Research: A Systematic Review." *Frontiers in sports and active living* vol. 4 860356. 25 Mar. 2022, doi:10.3389/fspor.2022.860356.

Mah, Cheri D et al. "The effects of sleep extension on the athletic performance of collegiate basketball players." *Sleep* vol. 34,7 943–50. 1 Jul. 2011, doi:10.5665/SLEEP.1132.

Schwartz, Jennifer, and Richard D Simon Jr. "Sleep extension improves serving accuracy: A study with college varsity tennis players." *Physiology & behavior* vol. 151 (2015): 541–4. doi:10.1016/j.physbeh.2015.08.035.

Zumwalt, M. (2018) *The Exercising Female.* Routledge.

About the Author

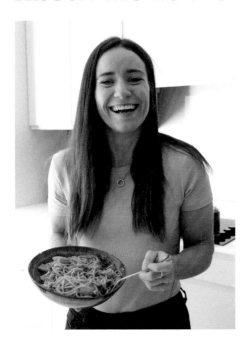

Laura Kealy is a health and performance nutritionist with more than ten years of experience working with female team sport athletes. She holds a Master of Science in Human Nutrition from the University of Ulster and a Postgraduate Degree in Sport and Exercise Nutrition from Leeds Beckett University. Laura is also registered with the Association of Nutrition (ANutr) and the Sports and Exercise Nutrition Register (SENr). Since founding her company Bridge Nutrition in 2018, Laura has supported hundreds of female athletes, both amateur and elite, across a range of sports. Laura currently resides in Dublin, Ireland, and supports both local and international athletes. In her spare time, Laura enjoys playing Gaelic football with her local team, trips in her camper van and adventure races with her brothers.

Follow Laura online:

Bridgenutrition.ie

 @bridgenutrition

 @laurakealybridgenutrition

Recipe Index

Credits

Cover design: Annika Naas
Interior design: Anja Elsen
Layout: DiTech Publishing Services, www.ditechpubs.com
Cover photo: © AdobeStock
Interior stock images: © AdobeStock
Interior photos: © Meyer & Meyer Sport (UK) Ltd.
Photographers: Luke Adams; Cara Gaynor
Illustrator: Madeleine O'Donnell
Managing editor: Elizabeth Evans
Copy editor: Sarah Tomblin, www.sarahtomblinediting.com